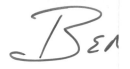

DRUGS & PERFORMANCE IN SPORTS

Edited by

RICHARD H. STRAUSS, M.D.

Associate Professor of Preventive Medicine and Internal Medicine, and Team Physician, Ohio State University, Columbus, Ohio

Associate Clinical Professor of Physiology, University of Hawaii School of Medicine, Honolulu, Hawaii

Philadelphia
London
Toronto
Mexico City
Rio de Janeiro
Sydney
Tokyo
Hong Kong

1987

W. B. SAUNDERS COMPANY

W. B. Saunders Company: West Washington Square
                           Philadelphia, PA 19105

Library of Congress Cataloging-in-Publication Data

Drugs & performance in sports.

1. Doping in sports.   I. Strauss, Richard H.   II. Title: Drugs
and performance in sports.

RC1230.D78   1987   615'.7   86–17770

ISBN 0–7216–1865–0

Acquisition Editor: Diana McAninch

Production Manager: Frank Polizzano

Manuscript Editor: June Gomez

Illustration Coordinator: Kenneth Green

Indexer: Joyce Anderson

Drugs and Performance in Sports   ISBN   0–7216–1865–0

Last digit is the print number: 9   8   7   6   5   4   3   2   1

CONTRIBUTORS

PER-OLOF ÅSTRAND, M.D.

Professor and Head, Department of Physiology III, Karolinska Institute, Stockholm, Sweden.

Why are Sports Records Improving?

ANDERS BORGSTRÖM

National Coach, Swedish Amateur Athletic Association, Karlstad, Sweden.

Why are Sports Records Improving?

DON H. CATLIN, M.D.

Associate Professor of Medicine and Pharmacology, University of California, Los Angeles, School of Medicine; Director, Paul Ziffren Olympic Analytical Laboratory, Los Angeles, California.

Detection of Drug Use by Athletes

TIMOTHY JON CURRY, Ph.D.

Associate Professor of Sociology, Ohio State University, Columbus, Ohio.

Magic, Science, and Drugs

ROD K. DISHMAN, Ph.D.

Associate Professor and Director, Behavioral Fitness Laboratory, Department of Physical Education, The University of Georgia, Athens, Georgia.

Psychological Aids to Performance

BJÖRN EKBLOM, M.D.

Professor, School of Physical Education, Karolinska Institute, Stockholm, Sweden.

Blood Doping, Oxygen Breathing, and Altitude Training

ARTHUR L. HECKER, Ph.D.

Adjunct Professor, Exercise Physiology, Ohio State University; Director, Medical Nutritional Research, Ross Laboratories, Columbus, Ohio.

Nutrition and Physical Performance

ZEBULON KENDRICK, Ph.D.

Associate Professor, Temple University School of Medicine and HPERD College, Temple University, Philadelphia, Pennsylvania.

Drugs, Exercise, and the Cardiovascular System

JOHN A. LOMBARDO, M.D.

Medical Director, Section of Sports Medicine, Cleveland Clinic Foundation, Cleveland, Ohio.

Stimulants; Depressants

DAVID T. LOWENTHAL, M.D., Ph.D.

Professor of Medicine and Pharmacology, Hahnemann University School of Medicine; Director of Clinical Pharmacology and Cardiac Fitness, Hahnemann Hospital, Philadelphia, Pennsylvania.

Drugs, Exercise, and the Cardiovascular System

THOMAS H. MURRAY, Ph.D.

Professor, Ethics and Public Policy, Institute for the Medical Humanities, University of Texas Medical School at Galveston, Galveston, Texas.

The Ethics of Drugs in Sports

ESTHER PARAN, M.D.

Associate Professor of Medicine, Soroka Medical Center, Ben Gurion University of the Negev, Beersheva, Israel.

Drugs, Exercise, and the Cardiovascular System

JONATHAN PARMET, M.D.

Resident in Medicine, Hahnemann University School of Medicine, Philadelphia, Pennsylvania.

Drugs, Exercise, and the Cardiovascular System

CARL L. STANITSKI, M.D.

Associate Clinical Professor of Orthopaedic Surgery, University of Pittsburgh School of Medicine; Staff Physician, Children's Hospital, Western Pennsylvania Hospital, and St. Margaret's Hospital, Pittsburgh, Pennsylvania.

Pharmacological Adjuncts to the Management of Musculoskeletal Injuries in Sports

RICHARD H. STRAUSS, M.D.

Associate Professor of Preventive Medicine and Internal Medicine, and Team Physician, Ohio State University, Columbus, Ohio; Associate Clinical Professor of Physiology, University of Hawaii, Honolulu, Hawaii.

Magic, Science, and Drugs; Anabolic Steroids; Effects of Therapeutic Drugs on Sports Performance

PREFACE

We live in a society in which drugs are widely used for the treatment of disease. Both prescription and nonprescription medications have helped to ease pain, improve function, and save lives in millions of people. Yet there is evidence that we are also an overmedicated society. It is not surprising, then, that athletes sometimes consider adding drugs to their training regimens in an attempt to improve performance beyond "normal" limits.

Which drugs—if any—enhance performance, and under what conditions? Are there harmful side effects? What are the ethical implications? Which drugs impair performance? These and other questions are answered by experts in each field.

This book is written for physicians whose patients are active in sports and therefore may be exposed to such drug use. The information is also of value to athletic trainers, nurses, coaches, and the athletes themselves.

The first section of the book deals with drugs and their perceived or real enhancement of athletic performance. Anabolic steroids, stimulants (including caffeine and cocaine), depressants (including marijuana), and blood doping are discussed. Drug testing and the ethics of drug use each comprise a chapter. Optimal nutrition and psychological aids that provide alternative methods for enhancing athletic performance are examined in detail.

The second section of this book discusses the effects of therapeutic drugs on active individuals—especially on their musculoskeletal and cardiovascular systems. Some therapeutic drugs, in addition to their primary action, affect sports performance adversely, and these side effects are also discussed.

At a time when drug use by athletes is frequently in the news, it is important for physicians and other health professionals to have ready access to the medical and scientific information about such use. It is hoped that this volume will help fill the need.

RICHARD H. STRAUSS

CONTENTS

I

ENHANCEMENT OF ATHLETIC PERFORMANCE

1

MAGIC, SCIENCE, AND DRUGS

RICHARD H. STRAUSS, M.D.
TIMOTHY J. CURRY, Ph.D.

A Fable

Long ago when the world was flat, a young Indian male—almost a brave—walked noiselessly in the vast forest of what we now call North America. Far ahead, he glimpsed a flash of bright orange as a Monarch butterfly darted through a narrow ray of summer sunlight that had edged between the canopied leaves. Already skilled with the bow and arrow, the young hunter had been told by the medicine man how to improve his speed and agility. He needed the butterfly. It was the first of the summer and would carry him far.

The lithe figure sprinted to the spot of sunlight but found no quarry. To his right, the forest brightened as it thinned and opened into a large meadow. It is there that the Monarch would have flown, to dry its wings in the open spaces. The Indian walked to the edge of the trees and looked across the meadow.

Twenty yards away the butterfly rested, fanning its orange and black wings slowly in the sun. Through its multi-faceted eyes it saw a crouching shape emerge noiselessly from the dark background of the woods. As the predator approached, its image grew larger and more threatening until, almost by reflex, the butterfly launched itself in the opposite direction, across the meadow and high into the sky where earth-bound creatures could never reach.

The hunter-athlete grunted in frustration but had no intention of giving up. He let the Monarch distance itself from him, then loped across the field, keeping it in sight. After a few minutes the butterfly felt safe, perhaps a bit tired, and landed in the grass. Again the Indian approached, this time crouching

3

lower, nearly crawling. And again the butterfly escaped. For twenty minutes the hunter ran, crouched, jumped, and ran again, finally catching the fragile creature between his cupped hands—in mid-air as its flight dipped carelessly close to earth.

The young man pressed a still-trembling wing between his thumb and finger. A thick coat of golden dust clung to his finger tips. He faced the strong morning sun and rubbed one wing of the butterfly across his bare chest. The magic dust mixed with the sweat of his pursuit. The medicine man had warned that it must be so for the butterfly to work its spell. As the almost-brave rubbed every trace of dust from the wings onto his skin, he knew that he had captured the darting speed of the Monarch. He would be the swiftest in his village.[1]

THE MAGIC OF DRUGS

Why do athletes use drugs? Because they believe that their performance will be improved, and occasionally this may be the case. But a major factor, which is usually ignored, is the placebo effect. *Placebo* is Latin for "I please." This effect has long been recognized as part of the magic in medicine. Many treatments that have no physiological effect still make the patient feel better. In sports, almost every coach and athlete agrees that psychological factors, such as self-confidence and the will to win, play an enormous role in determining the outer limits of performance. The pregame pep-talk is applied psychology, as is any treatment—whether a massage or an injection—that the athlete believes will help. If competitors think they will perform better, they probably will.

Magic is unnecessary when one can completely control a situation, or at least can predict the outcome with certainty. However, superstition and ritual—wearing certain socks or eating a Big Mac before the game—may become important when the results are unpredictable and the athlete needs a little bit of luck.[2] Then magic can't hurt, and it might even help. The problem with drugs is not their magic, but their side effects. Some of them *can* hurt.

SCIENCE AND DRUGS

The biological effects of drugs on athletic performance are difficult to study scientifically for several reasons. Scientists do well to observe changes of 5 per cent, yet races are won by a fraction of 1 per cent. The placebo effect must be neutralized by making sure that neither the athlete being tested nor the scientist making the observations knows whether the drug that was administered was the real thing or an inert fake. Other influences on performance, such as fatigue, nutrition, and motivation, must be kept as constant as possible. The number of trials must be large enough to result in statistically significant results.

Of course, these problems are part of many scientific studies. The real problem is that most drugs used in sports, particularly in the large doses currently employed, are known to have at least some harmful effects. And most scientists, or the ethics committee to whom they report, are unwilling to subject people to these known risks. As a result, it is difficult to perform scientifically sound experiments. We rely largely on older studies that used small doses of drugs or on uncontrolled observations of athletes who are administering drugs to themselves.

PATTERNS OF DRUG USE IN SPORTS

For thousands of years, athletes and warriors have used diverse substances in an attempt to improve their physical performance. Whether rubbed on the skin or ingested, most purported aids to performance have no physiological effect and, therefore, live and die as fads that last only long enough to be recognized as useless. However, a few substances have been shown scientifically to enhance or degrade performance, and it is these that are discussed in this book.

Ancient Greek athletes and modern high-school football players often have maintained that eating meat improves sports performance. It is true that meat—or at least high-quality protein—is necessary for good nutrition, but how much? In a society that has insufficient dietary protein, additional meat fed to athletes could, in fact, aid performance by improving nutrition to adequate levels. But a meal of steak shortly before a football game can be counterproductive, because protein and fat remain in the stomach for a considerable time and do not contribute to the energy requirements of the game.

The use of drugs to alter performance seems to have originated in both sport and combat situations. The ancient Romans punished manipulation of race horses before the race, it being said the culprits were subject to crucifixion.[3] The word *assassin* stems from *hashshashin*, those who habitually used hashish with its high concentration of tetrahydrocannabinol, the active ingredient of marijuana. In the Middle Ages, assassins were Muslim fanatics whose chief goal was to kill crusaders.[4] In World War II, a small number of German soldiers took newly developed anabolic-androgen steroid hormones in an attempt to increase their aggressiveness in combat,[5] and American soldiers were given the stimulant amphetamine to improve their endurance and attentiveness when deprived of sleep.[6] American soldiers brought the use of amphetamines back to their postwar activities as truck drivers, college students, and athletes.

Amphetamines became popular among bicycle racers in lengthy competitions and were associated with several deaths in the 1960 Olympic Games and in the 1967 Tour de France.[7] Amphetamines have been used by weight lifters, football players,[8] and other athletes in the hope of improving speed, strength, endurance, or aggressiveness.[9] Cocaine and caffeine have been used as stimulants for centuries by South American Indians.[10] Reports of abuse of cocaine by modern athletes are widespread.

Strychnine also stimulates the central nervous system and was used for a limited period by prize fighters.[7] The main problem is that the dose of strychnine that causes mild central nervous system stimulation is only slightly less than the dose that causes convulsions and death.

The term *doping* originated in South Africa, where *dop* was the name of an alcoholic beverage used by a native population.[3] Currently, doping refers to the use of drugs or other substances in an attempt to enhance the performance of humans, racehorses, or other animals. Blood doping is the infusion of additional blood into an athlete—their own blood or another person's—in an attempt to improve endurance. It has been used by Olympic athletes,[11] although it is now considered unethical and is banned by the International Olympic Committee.

Anabolic-androgenic steroid hormones are synthetic male hormones that are related to the natural male hormone, testosterone. It is thought that they were first used in Olympic competition in 1960 in an attempt to increase strength.[12] Initially, anabolic steroids were used by male competitors in sports requiring great strength, such as shot put, discus throw, javelin, and weight lifting. However, their use has spread widely. At international competitions where drug testing is performed, anabolic steroids have been detected among men competing in wrestling and distance running, as well as in the strength sports.[13] Women competing in shot put, discus throw, running, and the pentathlon also have been found to be using anabolic steroids.[12]

The use of drugs as performance aids is widespread not only at the international level but has also filtered down to include some or many athletes—depending on the sport—at national, college, and even high-school levels, as well as in the professional ranks.[14]

THE ATHLETE'S DILEMMA

The founder of the modern Olympics, Baron Pierre de Coubertin, said in 1908: "The important thing in the Olympic Games is not to win but to take part; the important thing in life is not the triumph but the struggle. The essential thing is not to have conquered but to have fought well."[15] Still, winning appears to be significant to many people. Perhaps the following statement is more applicable these days: "In the Olympics you cannot just be beaten and then depart, but first of all, you will be disgraced not only before the people of Athens or Sparta or Nicopolis but before the whole world. In the second place, if you withdraw without sufficient reason you will be whipped. And this whipping comes after your training, which involves thirst and broiling heat and swallowing handfuls of sand" (Epictetus, ca. 120 A.D.).

On one hand, there is great social pressure for the athlete to win at all costs, whether the contest is a high-school basketball game or an Olympic 100-meter dash. On the other hand, participants are supposed to follow certain rules in competing, such as not taking a short cut in the marathon. Drugs as aids to sports performance are disapproved by most of the population of the world for several reasons: (1) drugs are artificial, potentially dangerous, and not part of the nature of sport; and (2) parents do not want children to find out that their heroes are using drugs, whether the drugs are anabolic steroids, cocaine, or marijuana (Fig. 1).

The immediate pressures to win are stronger for many athletes than the admonition not to use drugs. Potential dangers are remote (everyone under 35 years old thinks that he or she is immortal), while victory is today's problem. "Taking medications to improve performance when you are sick with an infection or pain is common; why not use them when healthy? All your competitors are on drugs, so you need them to stay even." Drugs are readily available to athletes throughout the world. Thus, the decision—whether to use them or not—is essentially up to the athlete.

Encouragement to use performance-related drugs may emanate from those with a vested interest in the athlete's winning, although not necessarily in his long-term well-being. The team or organization shares the athlete's desire for victory, or else it would go out of business.

Berry's World

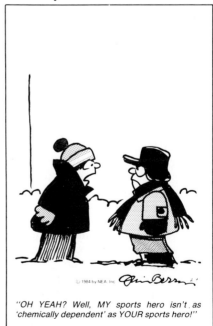

Figure 1–1. © 1984 Newspaper Enterprise Association, Inc.

"OH YEAH? Well, MY sports hero isn't as 'chemically dependent' as YOUR sports hero!"

Occasionally parents seek growth hormone to make their child a taller basketball player or bigger football player and increase his or her chances of getting a college scholarship.

DETERRING DRUG USE

Should drugs be banned in sports? No, say some competitors. They feel that their bodies are their own, to do with what they wish without interference from paternalistic organizations. If they play football, they run an increased risk of injuring their knees for life, so they'll accept a small possibility of liver cancer with anabolic steroids. They believe that the prohibition of drugs in sports is as futile as the prohibition of alcohol was in the United States.

In contrast, world opinion and most sports organizations feel that drug use should be controlled. But how? The following techniques are employed.

1. *Control the supply. Make it impossible for athletes to obtain drugs.* Apparently this does not work. Most athletes can get the drugs they want. Money may or may not be part of the trade. This applies at least to upper level competitors throughout the world, local laws notwithstanding.

2. *Education.* Partly effective. Many athletes who learn about both the performance and harmful effects of drugs choose not to use them.

3. *Testing.* Partly effective. The use of stimulants, such as amphetamine and cocaine, essentially has been eliminated at contests in which testing is done. This is because stimulants must be taken within a few hours of the contest to have a physiological effect and are, therefore, easily detected in urine.

Anabolic steroids are a different story. The oil-based injectables can be detected for months after use, so athletes who know that they will be tested stay away from these substances. The oral anabolic steroids can be detected for a variable number of weeks, so the game becomes one of cops and robbers. A few nations test top athletes at unannounced times. This probably is effective in deterring the use of drugs that are detectable in urine, but it raises questions of civil liberties in the minds of some. In such countries, athletes argue that they are at a disadvantage compared to nations that do not test randomly or fail to ban competitors found to be using drugs. Currently, there is no test for growth hormone, blood doping, or certain other substances.

Drug testing is expensive and can be performed at only a limited number of contests or on limited groups of athletes. For the vast number of sports participants—the young and those who have not reached the conspicuous top of the heap—education about the negative effects of performance drugs is an important deterrent.

AHEAD IN THIS BOOK

Factors that help or hinder athletic performance are discussed in greater detail in the following chapters. They include physical and physiological contributions to improving sports records; optimization of nutrition; psychological aids; anabolic steroids; stimulants, depressants, and blood doping; drug detection; and the ethics of drugs in sports.

Drugs are, of course, used widely for the treatment of injuries and illnesses among athletes, just as in the general population. Such use is intended to bring the athlete up to his or her normal, healthy level of performance. The second section of this book covers drugs used in the treatment of musculoskeletal trauma, cardiovascular abnormalities, and diseases such as asthma, diabetes, and the common cold. It is clear that drugs or other aids to performance may be applied either wisely or unwisely in sports.

REFERENCES

1. This story is fictitious. It is based on the alleged use of the powder from butterfly wings in this manner by American Indians.
2. Eitzen DS, Sage GH: Sociology of American Sport. Dubuque, IA, William C Brown, 1982, pp 163–167.
3. Prokop L: The struggle against doping and its history. J Sports Med Phys Fitness 10:45–48, 1970.
4. Stein J (ed): The Random House Dictionary of the English Language. New York, Random House, 1967.
5. O'Shea JP: Anabolic steroids in sport: A biophysiological evaluation. Nutr Rep Int 17(6):607–627, 1978.
6. Cooter GR: Amphetamine use, physical activity and sport. J Drug Issues (summer): 323–330, 1980.
7. Thomason H: Drugs and the athlete. In Davies B, Thomas G (eds): Science and Sporting Performance: Management or Manipulation? Oxford, Oxford University Press, 1982, pp 100–110.
8. Mandell A: The Nightmare Season. New York, Random House, 1976.
9. Toohey JV: Non-medical drug use among intercollegiate athletes at five American universities. Bull Narcotics 30(3):61–64, 1978.
10. Hollyhock M: The application of drugs to modify human performance. Br J Sports Med 4:119–127, 1969.
11. Rostaing B, Sullivan R: Triumphs tainted with blood. Sports Illustrated 62(3[Jan 21]):12–17, 1985.
12. Shuer M: Steroids. Women's Sports 4(4[April]):17–23, 1982.
13. Cart J, Harvey R: Finland's Vainio forfeits silver medal after failing drug test. Los Angeles Times, August 13, 1984, p VIII–8.
14. Special report—Drug abuse in sports: Denial fuels the problem. Phys Sportsmed 10(4):114–123, 1982.
15. Henry B, Yeomans PH: An Approved History of the Olympic Games. Sherman Oaks, CA, Alfred Publishing Company, 1984, p ix.

2

THE ETHICS OF DRUGS IN SPORT

THOMAS H. MURRAY, Ph.D.

Athletes young and old are increasingly faced with a difficult choice: to use drugs or other performance aids or accept what amounts to a competitive handicap. It is a choice with significant ethical dimensions. Should athletes be permitted—or forced—to make this choice? Or should society, through the medium of sports governing bodies, take the decision away from the athletes by banning the use of drugs and effectively enforcing that ban?

If we say that the choice ought to be left to the athletes, we are opting to respect individual liberty over other ethical considerations. If, on the other hand, we choose to ban performance-enhancing drug use in sports, we are deciding to protect the athlete against the potentially harmful consequences of his or her own choices. In other words, we would be acting paternalistically. Paternalism, especially medical paternalism, has a bad reputation today. But it can be justified in particular circumstances. Is a prohibition of drugs in sports justified or unjustified paternalism?

Before trying to answer these questions directly, it might be useful to take a brief look at the history of drug use in sports and at the concept of a "performance-enhancing drug."

HISTORY OF DRUG USE IN SPORTS

Reports of drug use, probably of mushrooms and herbs, date as far back as the ancient Greek Olympiads. We do not know what effect these ancient concoctions had, although we should not underestimate the psychological power of placebos. One modern Olympic athlete tells a story of a sprinter who, at the starting line, conspicuously placed a large tablet in her mouth. According to the story, the other runners were so perplexed at this that the one with the tablet won easily. The tablet was physiologically innocuous, although psychologically powerful—as gamesmanship. Some critics of modern drug use in sports believe that virtually all of the claimed effects of steroids and other drugs are nothing more than placebo effects.

By the late nineteenth century, coca leaf extracts (the source of cocaine) were widely available. A French product, Vin Mariani, which was a combination of wine and coca leaf extract, was even touted as the "wine for athletes." French cyclists used it, and so apparently did a championship lacrosse team. At that time, cocaine and coca leaf extract were not yet legally banned and indeed were celebrated by certain physicians and others as increasing one's energy and stamina. Bolivian Indians had long relied on chewing wads of coca leaf to help stave off hunger and fatigue caused by long hard hours of work.

Drugs probably entered the modern Olympics in the 1952 Oslo winter games where there were reports of used hypodermics and empty ampules in the athletes' locker rooms. It is likely that stimulants, quite possibly amphetamines, were used. By the early 1960's, the drug category of choice appears to have become the anabolic steroids. Events moved rapidly after that. Harold Connolly, who competed in several Olympics, told a committee of the U.S. Senate that "It was not unusual in 1968 to see athletes with their own medical kits, practically a doctor's, in which they would have syringes and all their various drugs. . . . I know any number of athletes on the 1968 Olympic team who had so much scar tissue and so many puncture holes in their backsides that it was difficult to find a fresh spot to give them a new shot."[1]

Anabolic steroid use probably began among elite male athletes whose events required lifting or throwing weights. By 1976, use by elite female athletes was widely suspected. In that year, women on the East German swimming team in Montreal were notorious for their masculine features and bass voices. Their coach's defense was classic: "We have come here to swim, not sing."[2]

In some events, steroid use was probably epidemic by the late 1970's. George Frenn, an Olympian competing in the hammer throw, said "I honestly cannot name one guy, and I know just about all of them personally, who is not using steroids." Furthermore, both the population of users and the doses taken had grown. Harold Connolly, speaking for the generation of Olympians who began competing in the 1960's, said "Athletes now are taking doses that would have blown our minds, and kids are taking them younger."[1]

Use of performance-enhancing drugs was not limited to elite amateur athletes. In the mid-1970's came word of team-sanctioned amphetamine use by professional football players. According to one NFL veteran, the first question asked of an injured player was "What else have you taken today?" Codeine-based painkillers may also have been used commonly, and there are reports of steroid use as well. Professional baseball seems to have been less hospitable to performance-enhancing drug use, although one journalist claims that the old Washington Senators team used to keep a cereal bowl of amphetamines available for its players.[3] Since then, there have been suggestions that younger, less skilled athletes are also using drugs such as steroids. The dimensions of the problem have grown considerably larger.

THE IDEA OF A PERFORMANCE-ENHANCING DRUG

Drugs appear to have entered sports in a major way only in the last 20 years or so. Official reaction to them has been inconsistent. Sports officials voice unequivocal disapproval of performance-enhancing drugs and formally ban them. Yet, when violations are uncovered, punishment is inconsistent. And there is growing evidence that use of banned performance aids is tolerated, and perhaps even encouraged, by some coaches, trainers, and physicians.

Part of the uncertainty in the response to performance-enhancing drug use in sports has been due to confusion about what the concept of a "performance-enhancing drug" really means. Confusion about the moral grounds for prohibiting the use of such drugs in athletic competitions also contributes to the uncertain reaction.

There are several reasons why the concept of a performance-enhancing drug is confusing. First, it is difficult even to define clearly what we mean by "drug." Some cases are easy and obvious. We can agree that heroin and penicillin are drugs, although very different from one another. But what about caffeine? It is freely available in coffee, soft drinks, and chocolates. We are accustomed to thinking of drugs as things that properly belong under the control of physicians. Caffeine escapes medical control, as do a host of over-the-counter drugs, so it cannot be medical control alone that allows us to identify something as a drug.

Is it that drugs have clear physiological effects? Certainly that would include caffeine and alcohol, as well as all or most prescription drugs. But does that mean we must include sugar? (For parents who have seen the impact of large doses of sugar on their young children, there can be no doubt about its physiological potency.) By itself, physiological effect cannot distinguish things we call drugs from some foods, or even from other things that influence our physiology, such as depressing events or sexual stimulation.

Perhaps the best definition of a drug is a tongue-in-cheek definition currently circulating among researchers—"a drug is any substance that, injected into a rat, produces a scientific paper." In reality, we do not need a perfect definition of "drug" to be able to distinguish, most of the time, between drugs and nondrugs. It is important, though, to note that a substance need not be under physicians' control to be classified legitimately as a drug. Consistent with that, the International Olympic

Committee has chosen to regard high levels of caffeine in the body as a violation of its anti-"doping" rules.

In any case, drugs are not the only source of performance enhancement that raises ethical problems. Blood packing, for one, involves the use of medical techniques but not the administration of drugs.

Another important point is that not all uses of drugs to enhance performance are regarded as wrong. For example, we would not object to a diabetic athlete injecting insulin. Nor would we see anything wrong in an athlete using an antibiotic to treat a bacterial infection. Finally, we do not even mind if an athlete takes a drug for symptomatic relief of a common cold, so long as the drug does not act as a central nervous system stimulant or otherwise go beyond the permissible goal of restoring normal health to the questionable goal of conferring a supranormal advantage.

Rightly or wrongly, most of us believe that there is a sensible and important distinction between using a drug to restore normal health and using one to go beyond normality. Is that a reasonable way to think about this issue, or merely irrational sentimentality?

WHAT IS WRONG WITH PERFORMANCE-ENHANCING DRUG USE?

It would help if we could identify just what it is that bothers us about the use of drugs and other performance aids. It cannot be merely that by taking a drug an athlete's performance is improved. That is certainly true of the insulin-using diabetic, and yet we have no qualms about permitting that sort of drug use. Nor can our objection be to the fact that a drug was used. We object to performance aids that are not drugs, and as the example of the diabetic shows, we do not object to all drug use, even when it has an impact on performance. So what is the source of our objection to drugs like anabolic steroids, amphetamines, and human growth hormone and to other performance aids? The answer is almost obviously simple, yet it requires a complex view of the nature of sports.

ETHICS AND THE NATURE OF SPORTS

Competition, preferably fierce competition, and excellence are the watchwords of sports. But anyone who has tried to watch a sport with which they are unfamiliar—cricket is a good example for most Americans—realizes that one cannot make sense out of what is going on without first understanding the goals of the particular sport and the rules governing it. At the other extreme, a deep appreciation of the finer points of play and of the history of the sport greatly enhances our understanding and enjoyment as participants or spectators. The point here is that particular sports make sense only against the background of a shared understanding of how excellence is judged for that sport.

Most of us would agree, I suspect, that the common element in sports is the goal of identifying and rewarding certain forms of human excellence. This is explicit in the Olympic motto: "Higher, faster, stronger." Just as clearly, we regard some ways of attaining excellence as legitimate and important, others as trivial or illegitimate. Ability, effort, skilled coaching, strategic cunning, and teamwork are all positively regarded. Seeking unfair advantages, sabotaging competitors, and using banned equipment are seen as negative. It is in the very nature of sports that we choose the kinds of excellence to be prized and rewarded, and we make choices about what constitutes legitimate and illegitimate means of attaining those ends.

We give expression to those goals through the rules we set for a sport. The rules lay out the general conditions under which competition takes place. They prescribe, for example, the dimensions of the playing area and the characteristics of allowable equipment. We define the rules to ensure that athletes compete under the same conditions. We hold most factors constant so that what differences do emerge are the ones we believe to be important and legitimate—the ones such as physical ability, training, and competitive savvy which comprise the excellences we wish to identify and honor.

From one point of view, the rules governing a particular sport may seem arbitrary and senseless. Why must a shot weigh 16 pounds? Why must there be five basketball players on the floor for each team? Why not four or six? There are two answers to such questions. First, if we changed the shot to 12 pounds or 20 pounds for everyone, it would not be quite the same sport. Sometimes we do allow minor changes in the rules because we believe they will somehow improve the game; but we must recognize that they also change the sport, and we must be able to defend the change as one that preserves what is essential in the sport. The second answer is that if we allowed one team to have six or more players and limited the opponent to only five, we would be looking at the effect of sheer numbers rather than at the skills we believe good basketball teams exhibit. Both answers ultimately rely on a conception of what competition in each particular sport is designed to reveal: Which excellences are to be rewarded?

We keep coming back to the ideal of excellence and the purpose of sports as the encouragement and reward of excellence. If this is true, as I believe it is, then drugs and other performance aids should be banned because they do not reflect the forms of human excellence that sports are intended to honor. This judgment is as defensible as a comparable one to ban equipment that would unfairly advantage certain competitors or change the nature of a sport adversely. If we can defend banning jet-propelled running shoes or pogo stick poles for the pole vault, then we can also defend banning drugs and other performance aids on the grounds that they distort the nature of a sport and reward differences among competitors (such as the willingness to risk one's health by taking large doses of drugs) that are not among the forms of excellence we believe are important and relevant to the sport.

From this perspective, using performance-enhancing drugs and other performance aids is analogous to using lead-weighted bats in baseball or an underweight shot in the shot put. It is *not* like using advanced training methods or high-quality equipment. Actually, using drugs or other performance aids that increase the health risks of a sport is ethically worse than doctoring equipment. To understand why, let us look at what makes various forms of cheating in sports unethical.

Cheating in sports is unethical in several ways. First, it breaks the rules of the sport and, therefore, gives one competitor an unfair advantage over others. Second, cheating can rarely be accomplished without lying or immoral secrecy, and so a person who cheats also usually must lie to escape detection. Third, cheating can poison relationships among competitors and between competitors and officials, transforming what should be honest and positive social relationships into deceitful and mistrustful ones. Fourth, since cheating on any scale is usually discovered eventually, the trust and esteem in which athletes in that sport and athletics in general are held is damaged. On this last point, I believe that the image and integrity of the Olympics and international athletics in general have been damaged by revelations of widespread use of performance enhancers, such as the blood packing by U.S. Olympic cyclists and the use of steroids by weight lifters and strength athletes from many nations.

Beyond the unethical nature of cheating in athletics, there are additional moral problems with the use of drugs or similarly risky performance aids. First, drugs, like steroids or human growth hormone, introduce the possibility of long-term, poorly understood risks. We simply do not know, for example, what the long-term risks of liver disease or heart disease are for athletes taking massive doses of anabolic steroids. We are not sure any of these will occur, although studies of nonathletic populations who have used steroids for long periods (although at much lower doses) indicate the dangers may be significant.

In response to this, people like Norman Fost, who defends steroid use, argue that this concern is "paternalistic and disingenuous." It is paternalistic because "Adults have the right to decide what risks they will take, so long as they obey the law." It is disingenuous—insincere or lacking in candor—because "The incidence of serious harm from steroids appears to be low, but even if the figure were higher, it could not approach the incidence of disability from competitive sports" such as football or boxing.[4] These are strong charges, and unless they can be answered adequately, the case for banning steroids will be severely damaged. Can they be answered?

I think they can, based on an understanding of what actually goes on when athletes face the decision of whether to use steroids or similar performance aids. First, the charge of disingenuousness. It is true that we accept serious risks of harm in a number of sports, boxing and football being among the most risky. In fact, there are many people who believe that football and boxing, particularly at the professional level, are too

risky and ought to be banned or drastically altered. Many rule innovations—large penalties for "roughing" the quarterback and protective head
gear in amateur boxing—are explicitly intended to minimize the possibility of harm. Nonetheless, the nature of these two sports entails the
risk of harm: high-speed collisions in football, landing punches in boxing.
It would be hard to imagine eliminating the risks of contact or punching
in these sports, respectively, without changing them fundamentally.

Perhaps, then, we should ban football and boxing completely if all
we are concerned about is eliminating risk. But that is not our aim. We
propose to minimize those risks that are not part of the nature of the
sport. Steroids in football are an excellent example. There is nothing in
the nature of football that requires athletes to take steroids, and so the
risks of steroid use are unnecessary additions to the intrinsic risks of the
sport. To say that because some risks remain we have no business trying
to minimize unnecessary additional risk is like saying that because
people get hurt in auto accidents there is no point in providing safety
equipment like seat belts or in requiring people to wear them. The risk
of harm from a collision without a seat belt is much greater than the risk
of harm while wearing one. Just because we tolerate the risk of accidents
as an invariable part of traveling by car does not mean that we are
prohibited from doing other things to minimize the risk, such as enforcing
speed limits or seat belt laws.

What about the accusation that banning risky performance aids like
steroids is paternalistic? It clearly is paternalistic. The question is, "Is it
justifiable or unjustifiable paternalism?"

In a country where we place such great importance on individual
liberty and noninterference by authority, the charge of paternalism stings.
It makes good sense to require any rule-making body that wants to limit
liberty to make a strong case for its actions. In the case of steroids and
sports, there are two good responses to the charge of unjustified paternalism.

The first response is that the assumption that individual athletes
freely choose to use performance aids is a dubious one. Much of what is
known about the motivations of athletes who use performance aids
suggests that they feel trapped. An athlete who chooses to forego using
a performance aid when his or her competitors use it is surrendering a
competitive advantage. It is difficult to overestimate how important
success can become to an athlete, particularly athletes competing at the
elite level (although I hear reports of athletes at much lower levels and
at younger ages facing similar choices). When one has invested many
years of effort, suffered through countless hours of training, and given
up many other pursuits in life, even a slight margin of advantage can
seem enormously important. An athlete's efforts and self-esteem may be
so heavily invested in a sport that surrendering the edge to the competition might seem terribly painful. It is quite possible that, at the
beginning, the athlete did not know that the margin of success might
come down to a choice like this.

Most importantly, each individual athlete's dilemma is replicated in each of his or her competitors. If no athlete used a performance aid, no other athlete would have to do the same to keep up. When some use performance aids, then the others feel compelled to do the same or else surrender what might be the winning edge. If this sounds like a "drug" race comparable to the arms race, it should. It is a kind of "social trap" in which we are each the cause and the victim of our individual and collective actions. If we could effectively enforce a ban on performance aids, then athletes could compete confident in the knowledge that they were competing against other athletes and not someone else's pharmacy. So, the assumption that the choice to use performance aids is a fully free choice is grossly oversimplified and probably false.[5]

The second response to the charge of paternalism is that it is justified by the good it will do and the harm that will be avoided. Even if we grant that there should always be a presumption in favor of liberty and noninterference, we also must acknowledge that there are times when some restrictions on liberty really do no one a great disservice and, on balance, provide a considerable benefit to all. For instance, how many of us feel that our freedom has been seriously infringed because we are compelled by law to drive on the right side of the road (or on the left side in the United Kingdom)? No one is unfairly disadvantaged by such a rule, and we are all much better off without the regular prospect of head-on collisions with people who would prefer to drive on the left. Similarly, no athlete would be particularly disadvantaged, and all would be better off with an effective rule that banned the use of steroids.

On balance, the charge of unjustified paternalism is not warranted. For one thing, the coercive context of decisions to use performance aids makes it doubtful that the choices are free to begin with. For another, restrictions that have the effect of benefitting everyone without harming anyone may be justified, even if they do limit freedom somewhat, especially if it can be shown that, in the absence of the restriction, those who choose to use the performance aid are made worse off by their choice.

But decisions to ban the use of performance aids also carry costs, especially social costs created by unequal enforcement and the possibility of flagrant, widespread violations. Once we have decided that we are ethically justified in banning certain performance aids, we have to look at the costs of enforcement to determine if the cure may be worse than the disease. It is not irrational to believe that a practice such as steroid use is morally wrong, and yet decide that, on balance, a ban would cause more harm than good. We have to look at the specifics of drug use in sports to decide whether a ban is feasible.

IS A BAN ON PERFORMANCE AIDS FEASIBLE OR DESIRABLE?

Let us look at the costs of a ban on performance aids. First, detecting violations may be very difficult technically. For some drugs, such as the synthetic anabolic steroids, scientists have developed very sophisticated tests. But even these are not perfect and probably do not detect oral steroids taken a few weeks prior to testing. Since the enhancing properties of steroids operate during training rather than at the time of actual competition, athletes can avoid detection by discontinuing use at a safe interval before testing (if the time of testing is known beforehand, which in most of the world it is).

But not all performance-enhancing drugs are synthetic. Testosterone itself is the prototype anabolic steroid and is found in the normal human body. The detection problem then is more complicated: We must not merely detect the presence of the chemical, but must prove that it is present in unnatural quantity. Similarly, detecting blood-packing (if it is done with the athlete's own red blood cells) might require establishing that some abnormal level of a normal cell type exists. Comparable problems exist for human growth hormone. Detecting amphetamines is child's play compared to the problems encountered with many other performance aids. So, technical difficulties in detection raise one set of important, though not necessarily insurmountable, problems.

A second problem is cost. Sophisticated equipment and scientific expertise carry high price tags. The laboratory bill for testing at the 1984 Los Angeles Olympics was over one million dollars. What price is too high to curtail the use of drugs as performance aids? It is certainly likely that the tests for more common substances will come down in cost as procedures become automated and as experience generally enhances efficiency. But it is equally likely that new drugs will come along and that new methods of confounding existing tests will be discovered, requiring more complex—and expensive—tests and procedures.

A third problem is an ethical one—invasion of athletes' privacy by compelling them to submit urine or other samples for analysis. This is a serious consideration. But it must be placed in context alongside the much greater intrusions upon privacy that arise in the course of training, as coaches exhort, humiliate, and hover over every action and as trainers test, probe, prod, and manipulate. It appears that the invasion of privacy caused by the urine sample requirement pales in significance compared with the daily routine intrusions the elite athlete encounters.

A fourth problem is the competition that has already arisen between the athletes who use performance aids and the officials whose job it is to detect violations. The dodges athletes have employed to escape detection are too numerous to list and occasionally are ingenious. However, one story deserves telling here. A male athlete who used steroids voided his bladder before the test and, using a catheter, refilled his bladder with someone else's urine (his girlfriend's). Sure enough, the test showed no steroids; on the other hand, it revealed that he was pregnant. I have no way of knowing whether the story is true or apocryphal, but it illustrates the undeniable contest between athletes and testers.

A fifth problem is the ambivalence of enforcement authorities. Faced with the fact that detection is imperfect and uneven and that it is the naive athlete who is usually caught while many others, equally culpable, escape, authorities typically ban the athlete for "life"—only to reinstate the person within 18 months. The problem is further complicated by the suspicion that some nations—most Westerners suspect the Eastern European bloc—actively push the development and use of performance aids and even assist their athletes in evading detection. These accusations are impossible to prove or disprove, and some commentators suggest that the charges are little more than sour grapes on the part of Western athletes. But the likelihood of differences among nations in commitment to halting the use of illegitimate performance aids is real and troubling.

The sixth and last problem is the current scope of enforcement and its probable injustice. So far in the international Olympic movement, only the athletes themselves have been punished. Since it is likely that others besides the athletes knew of, tolerated, encouraged, or even demanded that the athletes use the banned performance aid—especially coaches, trainers, physicians, and officials of sports governing bodies—then these "others" are also guilty and equally deserving of punishment. It is unjust to punish only the athlete when many more people are involved. It is also probably ineffective in the long run.

These objections are important and deserve to be answered before establishing a policy of banning specific performance aids. Are the difficulties overwhelming? Should we allow performance aids in sports on the grounds that the costs of banning them are excessive? I do not think so.

While technically difficult, detection is not impossible for most performance aids. Where it is, other methods may be useful. For example, athletes in the pentathlon were suspected of using beta-blockers, which prolong the interval between heart beats. The pentathlon requires shooting, and athletes know that shooting between beats increases accuracy. Beta-blockers, by increasing the interval between beats, permit more time to aim and shoot. But beta-blockers may also have a negative effect on endurance. So one way of discouraging their use is to schedule an endurance event on the same day as the shooting event. Athletes would not gain any net advantage by using beta-blockers, since improved shooting scores would be offset by slower times in the running event.

Cost is a legitimate concern, and it makes sense to search for economies wherever possible. For one thing, random, unannounced testing for drugs like steroids or human growth hormone that must be taken over long periods of time to be effective is much more likely to be successful in discouraging their use and could even be less expensive.

I have discussed privacy above. The contest between testers and takers is a distressing feature of any ban and will not disappear completely so long as some athletes persist in trying to evade detection. One constructive approach would be to deal with the adversarial nature of the tester/official-athlete relationship by involving the athletes themselves in policy making. A fair and effective ban is in the athletes' interest and could be accomplished more efficiently and ethically with the cooperation of the athletes themselves in devising and carrying out policy. Any involvement on the part of athletes though must be substantial and genuine, not mere window dressing.

A general increase in fairness would go a long way toward solving the problem of effectiveness, as athletes would be more inclined to adhere to an equitable ban. One of the most important steps that must be taken is to lay sanctions on *all* the guilty parties, not merely the athlete. Coaches, trainers, and sports physicians have enormous influence over athletes and are in a position to discourage illegitimate performance aids. If they too were punished when athletes under their supervision are discovered to have violated the ban, they would have strong incentives to make certain their athletes were not defying the prohibition. Whether the people who govern national and international sports have the courage to extend sanctions to nonathletes remains to be seen.

CONCLUSION

Drugs and other performance aids raise a number of difficult ethical and policy questions. Performance aids that do not conform to our conception of what forms of human excellence are important to sports are forms of cheating and are unethical. Banning such aids would not be a form of unjustified paternalism, because (1) the choices of individual athletes are more coerced than free and (2) much good will come from an effective ban and much harm may be avoided. Devising and implementing a policy to ban illegitimate performance aids will be difficult and may run into a number of practical and ethical problems. In the case of drugs and other illegitimate performance aids in sports, a fair and effective policy of prohibition could probably be created, although there is reason to doubt whether current policies meet even the minimum requirements. There is no question that current policies could be improved substantially.

REFERENCES

1. Lorge B: A thoroughly modern athlete: Bigger, better—and on drugs. Washington Post, May 27, 1979, p A–6.
2. Amdur N: Mounting drug use afflicts sports world. New York Times, November 20, 1978, pp C–1, 8.
3. Boswell T: Number of "poppers" in baseball grows fewer each season. Washington Post, May 28, 1979, p D-4.
4. Fost N: Let 'em take steroids. New York Times, September 9, 1983, p A–19.
5. Murray TH: The coercive power of drugs in sports. Hastings Center Report, August, 1983, pp 24–30.

3

NUTRITION AND PHYSICAL PERFORMANCE

ARTHUR L. HECKER, Ph.D.

Dedication and creative training techniques are an athlete's most effective means of developing natural abilities. One component of training is optimal nutrition. Nutritional conditioning, like physical conditioning, is a continuous quest, not something to be practiced a day or two before competition. Top performance cannot happen if an athlete does not maintain an optimal nutritional regimen during the entire training and competitive season.

Nutritional factors can influence performance at every stage of training and competition. The four critical nutritional periods can be described as

1. Nutritional maintenance during training
2. Pre-event nutrition
3. Nutritional support during competition or training
4. Post-event or post-training nutrition

In this chapter, the physiological and biochemical research that has defined optimal nutrition during these critical periods will be discussed. Nutritional regimens for optimal training and performance will be outlined, and controversial practices will be discussed.

Portions of this chapter have been excerpted from Hecker AL: Nutritional conditioning for athletic competition. Clin Sports Med 3:567, 1984.

NUTRITIONAL MAINTENANCE DURING TRAINING

The most commonly ignored but most important period of an athlete's "nutritional" season is training. Because the ultimate competitive ability of a person is related to his or her capacity to train maximally, every effort must be made to ensure that all nutritional needs are met during this period. Proper nutritional management during training also supports the athlete during competition.

THE BASIC DIET

The diet of an athlete in training must contain appropriate amounts of all essential nutrients. Although no one diet is totally adequate for all athletes, a basic well-balanced diet can be tailored to meet specific needs. Simply stated, a nutritionally adequate diet provides sufficient nutrients (including water) and energy to meet metabolic needs for optimal functioning of the body. This basic diet should follow the Recommended Dietary Allowances (RDA), which take into account (1) the body's structural requirements, (2) the relative efficiency of various foods to serve as fuel, (3) the complex interactions of nutrients during digestion, and (4) current knowledge regarding long-term health factors.[51]

A basic diet can be designed utilizing the four basic food groups: (1) milk and milk products; (2) meat and high protein foods; (3) fruits and vegetables; and (4) cereal and grain foods. The minimal intake should

TABLE 3–1. Example of Basic Diet* (Low Caloric Intake)

	Calories
Breakfast	approximately 300
1/2 bowl cereal (Cheerios, corn flakes, Wheaties, raisin bran, etc.)	
1 cup milk (2% fat)	
1/2 piece toast (butter and jelly)	
1 cup orange juice	
Lunch	approximately 600
1-1/4 cup macaroni and cheese dinner (Kraft)	
1 banana	
1 granola bar	
1 cup milk (2% fat)	
Dinner	approximately 800
1-1/2 cups ravioli or spaghetti (canned or homemade with sauce)	
1 slice bread with butter	
1/2 cup applesauce	
2 cups milk (2% fat)	
1/2 cup pudding, chocolate, canned	
	Total Calories 1700

*Individual food preferences should be taken into account when selecting specific foods from the basic food groups. The composition of different foods can be obtained from Nutritive Value of American Foods. Agriculture Handbook 456, Agricultural Research Service, USDA, 1975.

TABLE 3–2. Example of Basic Diet* (High Caloric Intake)

	Calories
Breakfast	approximately 950
2 bowls cereal (Cheerios, corn flakes, etc.)	
2 cups milk (2% fat)	
2 pieces toast (butter and jelly)	
2 cups orange juice	
Lunch	approximately 1250
2-1/2 cups macaroni and cheese dinner (Kraft)	
1 cup applesauce	
1 granola bar	
1 cup milk (2% fat)	
Snack	approximately 350
1 doughnut (iced-cake)	
1 cup milk (2% fat)	
1 apple	
Dinner	approximately 1450
6 pancakes (syrup and butter)	
2 eggs	
2 cups milk (2% fat)	
1 cup orange juice	
1 banana	
1 pudding (4 oz)	
	Total Calories 4000

*Individual food preferences should be taken into account when selecting specific foods from the basic food groups. The composition of different foods can be obtained from Nutritive Value of American Foods. Agriculture Handbook 456, Agricultural Research Service, USDA, 1975.

include two servings per day from the milk group, two from the protein-rich group, and four from the cereal/fruit/vegetable groups.[56] Table 3–1 describes a basic diet developed in accordance with these principles. This regimen will result in a caloric distribution of approximately 60 to 65 per cent from carbohydrate, 12 to 15 per cent from protein, and 25 to 30 per cent from fat. The food intake pattern can be adjusted for weight gain or loss, and for maintenance by adjusting calories until the desired daily total is reached. To add calories, extra servings of food from the four groups should be eaten and can be based on individual preferences. If caloric requirements are high (more than 3000 Calories per day), frequent snacking may be necessary. Snacks should be primarily carbohydrate.

If caloric requirements are very high (above 4000 Calories per day), a more aggressive meal pattern should be followed. Table 3–2 describes one such diet. The food selections described in both Tables 3–1 and 3–2 are designed to optimize carbohydrate intake at the expense of fat. It is difficult to maintain high carbohydrate intakes without careful dietary management. Even small portions of meat dishes can have a dramatic impact on total fat and protein intakes. This relationship is often overlooked by athletes.

Well-conditioned athletes should not have fluctuations in body weight; therefore, they must monitor their daily food intake to ensure that they are consuming an appropriate number of calories to maintain a stable body weight. A lean, well-trained athlete who does not take in enough calories will lose muscle mass when losing body weight because lean athletes have very little body fat available to lose.

Role of Carbohydrate During Training

Once the basic dietary needs of the athlete have been satisfied, specific nutrient intakes can be considered. In addition, the form and concentration of the nutrients and the timing of their administration should be planned because these aspects of nutrition can also influence performance. Because of the limited carbohydrate storage capability of the body (in muscle and liver) and the relative ease with which these stores can be changed by diet and/or training, it is important that athletes and their support personnel (coaches, trainers, physicians, dietitians, and others.) have a knowledge of the dynamics of carbohydrate metabolism. In general, athletes can best meet the demands of daily training by following a high-carbohydrate diet regimen that includes three balanced meals with between-meal snacks as needed to meet caloric demands.

The importance of muscle carbohydrate stores is shown in Figure 3–1.[5] Glycogen is a form of carbohydrate used by the muscles to fuel movement. Figure 3–1 shows that, as exercise progresses, muscle glycogen levels drop. Fatigue is highly correlated with muscle glycogen depletion. Figure 3–2 further documents the critical role of carbohydrate.[6] These data show that the higher the level of muscle glycogen when exercise starts, the greater the endurance of the athlete. The amount of

MUSCLE GLYCOGEN
mmo1 GLUCOSYL UNITS kg^{-1}

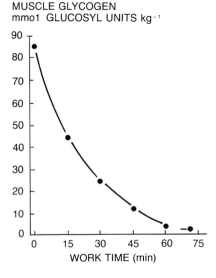

Figure 3–1. Muscle glycogen content during 75 minutes of cycling at 85 per cent of maximal oxygen uptake. (From Bergstrom J, Hultman E: The effect of exercise on muscle glycogen and electrolytes in normals. Int J Sports Med 1:3, 1980.)

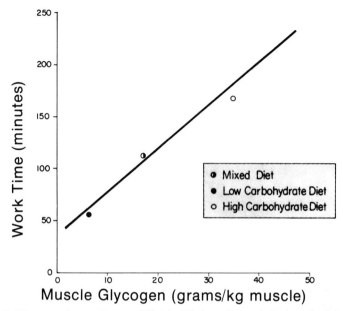

Figure 3–2. Effects are shown of a mixed ("normal") diet, a low carbohydrate (high fat) diet, and a high carbohydrate diet on the glycogen content of the quadriceps femoris and the duration of exercise on a bicycle ergometer. These data clearly show that the higher the initial level of muscle glycogen, the greater is the endurance capacity for submaximal exercise. (From Bergstrom J, Hermanson L, Hultman E, et al: Diet, muscle glycogen and physical performance. Acta Physiol Scand 71:140, 1967.)

carbohydrate in the diet has a dramatic effect on the initial concentration of glycogen in the muscle. Stores of glycogen in the liver also play a role in supporting exercise, but this role is not as critical as that of the muscle stores. The relationship between muscle and liver glycogen will be discussed later.

Hard physical training, especially twice-a-day workouts, can use up most of the glycogen stored in an athlete's muscles. If glycogen stores are not adequately replenished daily by the carbohydrate in the diet, the athlete will become chronically depleted. Chronic depletion of muscle glycogen leads to compromised performance (such as reduced speed, precision, and endurance). Chronic fatigue or "staleness" also may limit an athlete's ability to comply with a progressive training program and subsequently to compete at maximal potential.

The relationship between heavy training and muscle glycogen levels is illustrated in Figure 3–3.[15] When athletes had repeated daily exercise bouts, a low-carbohydrate diet allowed a declining cascade in muscle glycogen stores. In contrast, a high-carbohydrate regimen promoted a significant 24-hour glycogen rebound. Muscle glycogen levels returned nearly to normal by each succeeding day. According to the results shown in Figure 3–3, an athlete must consume 60 to 70 per cent of total calories

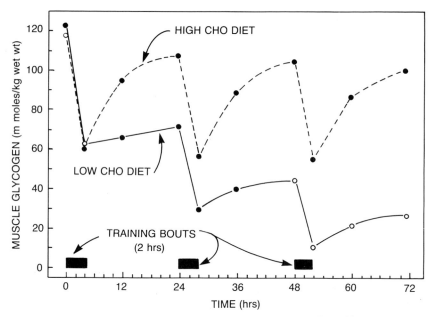

Figure 3–3. Muscle glycogen content is shown during three successive days of heavy training with diets whose caloric compositions were 40 per cent carbohydrate (low CHO) and 70 per cent carbohydrate (high CHO). (From Costill DL, Miller JM: Nutrition for endurance sport: Carbohydrate and fluid balance. Int J Sports Med 1:4, 1980.)

as carbohydrate to prevent chronic glycogen depletion. For a 3000 calorie diet, this would represent a total carbohydrate intake of approximately 1800 to 2100 calories (450 to 525 grams) per day.

The preceding effects of exercise on glycogen stores are not limited to muscle. Hultman and Nilsson used needle biopsies to demonstrate the same response in the liver (Fig. 3–4).[25, 36] Glycogen levels were measured after exercise, during several days of low-carbohydrate intake, and then after the resumption of a high-carbohydrate diet. Liver glycogen stores dropped significantly during exercise and fell even further during carbohydrate starvation. There was a dramatic rebound in liver glycogen levels after the introduction of a high-carbohydrate diet.

In addition to meeting carbohydrate-intake goals, an athlete also must consume enough total calories to meet the demands of the exercise program and to maintain a stable body weight. Athletes who are in a negative caloric balance compromise their ability to synthesize glycogen. Even elevated carbohydrate intake may not prevent chronic glycogen depletion if caloric intake is low. When caloric needs are not met, there is a risk that intakes of other nutrients may also be deficient, thus further limiting performance.

The form of the carbohydrate should also be considered when formulating a diet plan. Costill et al. have reported that the form of the

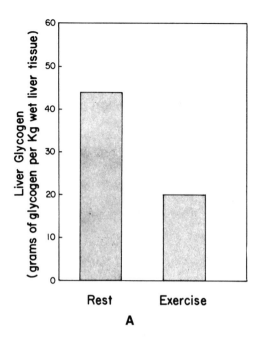

A

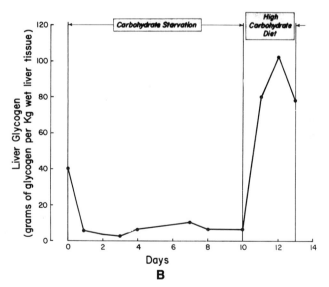

B

Figure 3–4. A, Liver glycogen is considerably reduced following exercise. B, There is a further reduction during several days of carbohydrate starvation. Note the overshoot, or supercompensation, one day after carbohydrate refeeding. (From Fox EL, Mathews DK: The Physiological Basis of Physical Education and Athletics, 3rd ed. Philadelphia, Saunders College Press, 1981.)

carbohydrate (that is, starch, glucose, sucrose, or fructose) had no significant effect on the rate of glycogen repletion during the first 24 hours following a heavy work bout (10 mile run at 80 per cent $\dot{V}_{O_2}$ max).[15, 16] This relationship is described in Figure 3–5. During the second 24 hours after the work bout, a diet rich in starches supported a greater ($p<0.05$) glycogen repletion rate than a diet rich in simple sugars. The reason for this delayed effect may be related to increased insulin sensitivity, because starch feedings maintain a prolonged insulin response compared with an equivalent glucose meal.[34] In addition, the activation of glycogen synthetase by insulin is well documented.[13] These data suggest that the practical needs of the athlete can be met by either a simple or complex carbohydrate source. Simple carbohydrates may be logistically more appropriate when an athlete participates in repetitive exercise (such as two-a-day workouts or tournament competition) or when the schedule of the athlete will not accommodate the time required to consume and digest meals containing complex carbohydrates.

Complex carbohydrates may be preferred on the basis of long-term health; however, there is no major concern about using simple carbohydrates occasionally. Exercise-trained individuals do not exhibit the same response to carbohydrate loads as sedentary subjects. For example, they demonstrate a lesser hyperglycemia and a lower insulin response to a given oral glucose load than do normally active subjects (Fig. 3–6).[15] Thus, these individuals have a greater tolerance of carbohydrate, diverting the majority of these calories to glycogen repletion with little impact on their serum lipid profile. For example, trained runners routinely exhibit serum triglyceride levels in the 40 mg/dl range even while on diets containing 70 per cent of total calories as mixed carbohydrates.[15]

Meal frequency sometimes can be a problem in designing a nutritional regimen. More frequent meals might be expected to support greater

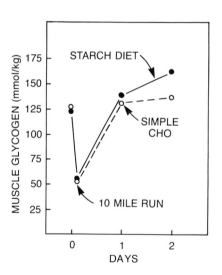

Figure 3–5. Influence of diets rich in starch and simple CHO (glucose, fructose, sucrose) on muscle glycogen restorage after exhaustive exercise. (From Costill DL, Miller, JM: Nutrition for endurance sport: Carbohydrate and fluid balance. Int J Sports Med 1:6, 1980.)

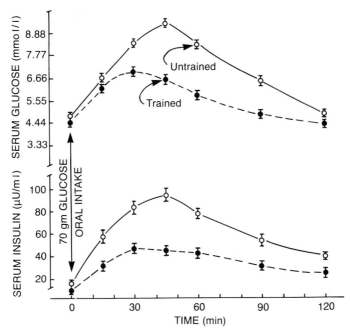

Figure 3–6. Oral glucose tolerance in endurance trained and untrained men. (From Costill DL, Miller JM: Nutrition for endurance sport: Carbohydrate and fluid balance. Int J Sports Med 1:6, 1980.)

glycogen repletion. However, the work of Costill et al. suggests that increased meal frequency may not be a critical issue.[16] Figure 3–7 shows that although high carbohydrate intakes (70 per cent vs. 50 per cent and 25 per cent of calories) enhanced glycogen synthesis, frequency of increased feedings did not. Seven feedings of a 70 per cent carbohydrate diet induced the same degree of repletion as a two-meal regimen. This study does not imply that athletes should attempt to consume their daily intake in only two meals. It suggests only that if circumstances dictate, glycogen stores can be maintained on as few as two meals a day. Regarding long-term health, this meal pattern should not be recommended for continued use. "Meal feeding" (i.e., consumption of infrequent, large meals) has been related to increased lipid synthesis, which may be of concern to even a well-trained athlete.[65]

Because muscle glycogen levels are so important to athletic performance and because these levels can be changed by the nutritional practices of the athlete, many athletes attempt to maximize levels of muscle glycogen by following a "loading" or "supercompensation" regimen. The complete regimen is illustrated in Figure 3–8, procedure 3. The regimen is initiated one week before competition. For the first two to three days, the athlete consumes a *mixed diet of predominantly fat and protein* containing only 100 grams of carbohydrate per day. During this same

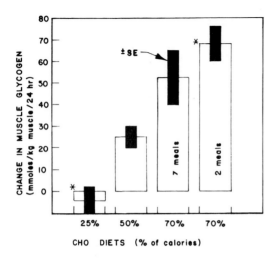

Figure 3–7. Effects of varied CHO diets on the restorage of muscle glycogen. Asterisk denotes a significant difference between that mean and the mean change in muscle glycogen observed during the mixed diet (50 per cent of calories from CHO). (From Costill DR, Sherman WM, Fink WJ, et al: The role of dietary carbohydrates in muscle glycogen resynthesis after strenuous running. Am J Clin Nutr 34:1831, 1981.)

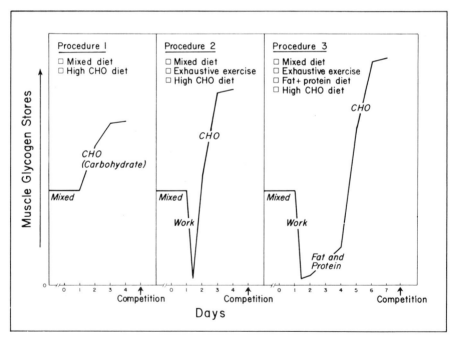

Figure 3–8. Glycogen loading procedures. (From Fox EL: Sports Physiology. Philadelphia, W.B. Saunders Company, 1979.)

period, an exhaustive training program is followed. For the remaining three to four days of the week, a high-carbohydrate (60 to 70 per cent of calories) diet is fed, and exercise is drastically reduced. The type of carbohydrate consumed during the glycogen loading regimen makes little difference to the rate and quantity of muscle glycogen stored. The result is a twofold or greater increase in muscle glycogen storage, which is localized in the exercising muscles.

A more moderate regimen is described by procedure 2 in Figure 3–8. This method omits the high-protein and high-fat dietary period but utilizes the exhaustive work schedule and high-carbohydrate dietary regimen. Some overcompensation can also be induced simply by increasing carbohydrate intake for three days before competition, omitting the initial depletion/heavy work phase of the regimen (Fig. 3–8, procedure 1). The latter procedure is adequate to meet the demands of training. Procedure 2 should be considered for pre-competition "loading."

The full glycogen supercompensation regimen should be used cautiously (if at all!) because of possible side effects. Electrocardiographic changes have been shown in at least one participant, and therefore glycogen loading may be potentially harmful for the individual who runs as a method of cardiac rehabilitation.[47] In addition, during the low-carbohydrate phase of the program, athletes find it difficult to train owing to fatigue associated with limited glycogen supplies. They are often irritable, and many experience decreased cognitive capabilities. Also, exhaustive training may not be warranted just before competition, as some athletes may suffer an injury or premature psychological/physiological peaking. The long-term health aspects of the high-fat and high-protein diets remain unresolved. Until more definitive data are available, it is recommended that these radical dietary alterations not be utilized on a weekly basis. Also, the full glycogen-loading regimen is not appropriate for young children. Youngsters involved in endurance activities should maintain optimal glycogen stores; however, the depletion phase of glycogen-loading should be omitted and only the repletion steps followed. Although carbohydrate consumption should be encouraged for all athletes, carbohydrate loading is most effective for long-term events such as soccer and endurance running.

Role of Fluids During Training

A critical nutrient for an athlete during any phase of training or competition is water. Most athletes are aware that acute fluid losses can be dangerous.[10, 51] What is often overlooked is that slight or moderate dehydration decreases exercise capacity (Fig. 3–9). Dehydration, particularly in combination with inadequate caloric intake, significantly reduces glycogen stores, endurance, power, and cognitive performance.[8, 34, 53]

Several investigators have reported that dehydration reduces the capacity of men to perform hard work, even in cool environments.[9, 12, 50, 52] The effect is most pronounced if dehydrated individuals attempt maximal competitive work in hot weather.[53] Dehydration is of particular concern in the weight-control sports, such as wrestling, boxing, and

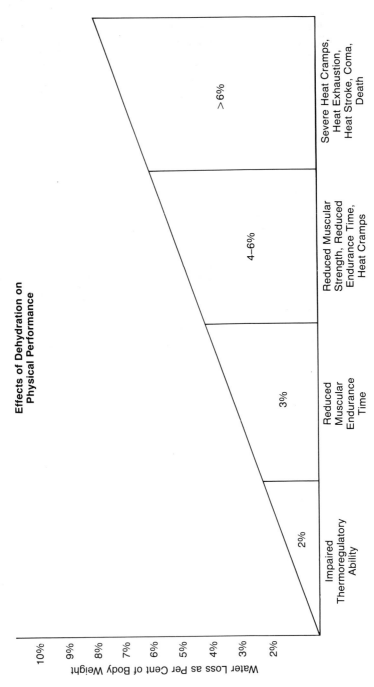

Figure 3–9. The relationship between fluid loss (per cent of total body weight) and physiological functions. (From Macaraeg PV, Santos CA: The effect of a glucose polymer electrolyte solution on exercise duration. National Athletic Trainers' Journal, Winter, 1984, p 263.)

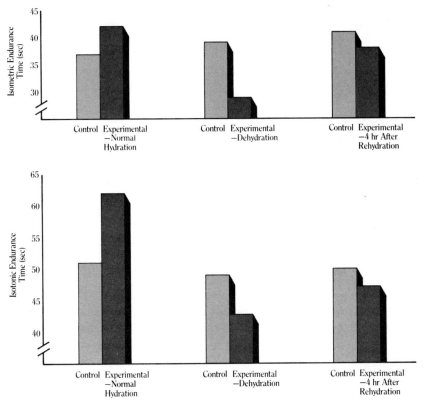

Figure 3–10. Change in muscular endurance time with dehydration (loss of 4 per cent body weight in water) and 4 hours after rehydration. The control group (10 people) received fluids throughout the study. The experimental group (also 10 people) was subjected to dehydration and rehydration. The large differences seen when both groups were normally hydrated are because of individual variation with these types of exercises. (From Torranin C, Smith DP, Byrd RJ: The effect of acute thermal dehydration and rapid rehydration on isometric and isotonic endurance. J Sports Med 19:1, 1979.)

light-weight crew. In these events, dehydration techniques are often used to achieve a lower weight classification. Figure 3–10 shows that following a 4 per cent loss of body weight from dehydration, muscular endurance time (averaged over all muscle groups) was 31 per cent shorter during isometric exercise and 29 per cent shorter during isotonic work.[59] Four hours after rehydration with a volume of fluid equal to the weight loss from dehydration, isometric and isotonic endurance times, respectively, were 13 per cent and 21 per cent below initial levels. Thus, not only was muscular endurance reduced by dehydration, but four hours was not sufficient time to restore normal muscular endurance. This contradicts the common assumption of weight-control competitors that four to five hours is an adequate amount of time to replace lost fluids.

TABLE 3–3. Concentrations of Glycogen, ATP, and CP in the Vastus Lateralis Muscles of Wrestlers* (Mean ± SEM for Wet-Tissue Weight)

Substrate	Diet Condition			
	C_1	D_1	D_2	R
Glycogen (mmole glucose units per kg)	62.3 ± 3.3	44.0 ± 3.0†	33.9 ± 1.8†‡	38.6 ± 2.7†
CP (mmole · kg^{-1})	19.4 ± 1.3	20.8 ± 0.3	21.4 ± 1.5	21.2 ± 0.8
ATP (mmole · kg^{-1})	5.8 ± 0.4	5.6 ± 0.3	5.1 ± 0.4	6.0 ± 0.5

*Before weight loss (C_1), after 48 hours of food intake reduction (D_1), after an additional 32 hours of food and liquid intake reduction (D_2), and after 3 hours of rehydration (R).
†Significantly less than C_1 (p<.05)
‡Significantly less than D_1 (p<.05)
From Houston ME, Marrin DA, Green JH, et al: The effect of rapid weight loss on physiological function in wrestlers. Phys Sports Med 9:73, 1981. Reprinted by permission of The Physician and Sports Medicine, a McGraw-Hill publication.

The combined effect of dehydration and food restriction was investigated by Houston et al.[35] The subjects (university wrestlers) reduced their body weight by 8 per cent using a combination of food restriction and reduced fluid intake. Table 3–3 describes the effect of the protocol on the amount of energy substrate in the muscle. Glycogen stores dropped dramatically by 48 hours and declined even further by the end of day three. The peak torque values for the individuals decreased as well (Fig. 3–11). It is important to note that here again the three-hour recovery period did not improve the glycogen levels or power.

Role of Thirst in Maintaining Hydration

Although thirst helps a resting person maintain water balance, it is an insensitive indicator of need for water in the athlete, especially one experiencing competitive anxiety. A resting person will maintain water balance by drinking enough water to satisfy thirst. Even in a hot environment, an unacclimatized person can come reasonably close to a stable fluid balance by just drinking to satisfy thirst. However, when a person begins to exercise, fluid loss escalates dramatically. As reported by Dill[20] and others,[1, 50] the thirst mechanism then will not compensate for fluid loss if the athlete works out every day. Even acclimatized men working in the heat never voluntarily drink as much water as they sweat.[1, 9, 50] In fact, they usually drink at a rate of about one half to two thirds the rate of loss. This suggests that to maintain fluid balance under these conditions requires that the exercise regimen be conducted on an every-other-day or even an every-third-day cycle. Not many athletes, or teams, are willing to accept a training program of such modest proportions (daily training is necessary to support optimal performance gains). Therefore, prevention of volunary dehydration requires aggressive fluid consumption. Athletes should weigh themselves before and after practice—any weight loss during this time can be assumed to be water. This

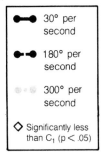

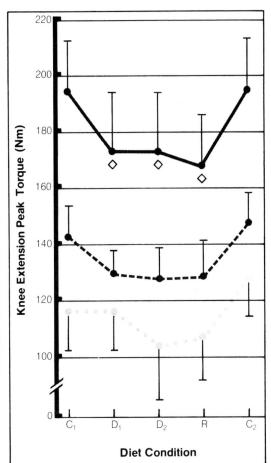

Figure 3–11. Peak torque values for wrestlers before weight loss (C_1), after 48 hours of food intake reduction (D_1), after an additional 32 hours of food and liquid intake reduction (D_2), after 3 hours of rehydration (R), and nine days after the completion of the experiment (C_2). Values are means with the standard error of the mean shown by the vertical lines. (From Houston ME, Marrin DA, Green HJ, et al: The effect of rapid weight loss on physiological function in wrestlers. Phys Sports Med 9:73, 1981. Reprinted by permission of The Physician and Sports Medicine, a McGraw-Hill publication.)

weight change, when added to normal requirements, can be used as an indicator of the actual quantity of fluid that should be consumed before the next training bout. As a safety precaution, any young athlete exhibiting more than a 2 per cent weight loss from day to day should be carefully monitored for symptoms of dehydration.

Role of Protein During Training

High protein intakes have never been shown to be beneficial to athletes.[64] Contrary to popular opinion, muscle size is not dependent on protein intake. If daily minimum protein intakes are met, muscle size will be dictated by the specific training program and, of course, genetic potential.

Protein metabolism increases with endurance exercise or vigorous strength training, but the impact of this increased turnover on protein requirements is not clear.[21] Protein requirements for athletes depend on the energy balance of the individual. This is illustrated by the study of Iyengar and Rao, who determined nitrogen balance in manual laborers on two energy intakes (44.4 and 55.5 calories per kilogram of body weight) and two protein intakes (1.0 and 1.2 grams per kilogram of body weight).[39] Men on low-energy intake plus low-protein intake (44.4 calories and 1.0 gram per kilogram) were found to be in negative nitrogen balance. However, positive nitrogen balance could be re-established by either increasing energy intake or increasing the protein intake.

Several studies have investigated whether the RDA of 0.8 gram per kilogram of body weight was adequate for athletes training under a variety of conditions and energy expenditures.[14, 30, 39, 44, 60] Table 3–4 shows that the RDA is sufficient for most work forms except perhaps during the initial phase of training. However, after adaptation to training, a neutral nitrogen balance is reestablished at a protein intake of 1 gram per kilogram of body weight. A self-selected diet will normally exceed this intake significantly. Such a diet will contain approximately 15 per cent of calories as protein. For an athlete consuming 4000 Calories per day, 15 per cent of calories represents 150 grams of protein, or 2.14 grams per kilogram for a 70 kilogram man. This is more than two and a half times the RDA. Even growing children in vigorous training programs will not require more than 1.5 grams per kilogram per day. Protein intakes exceeding the RDA are either burned for energy to support activity or are converted to fat. In addition, metabolism of excess protein results in residual nitrogen that must be discarded through the urine as urea. This step requires the loss of water, which can exacerbate an athlete's state of dehydration.

TABLE 3–4. Summary of Experiments Investigating the Sufficiency of the RDA Intake of Protein During Various Activities

Physical Activity	Protein Intake (gm/kg)	Energy Expenditure (kcal/kg)	Indicator of Protein Sufficiency	Reference
Manual labor	1.0	56	Positive nitrogen balance	Iyengar and Nageswara Rao[39]
Weight lifting (400 kcal/session)	0.8	68	Positive nitrogen balance	Marable et al.[44]
75 minutes of isometric exercises/day	1.0	50	Maintained body potassium (lean body mass)	Torun et al.[60]
Combination of several exercises	1.4	48	Positive nitrogen balance	Consolazio et al.[14]
Bicycle ergometer (start of training)	1.0	55	Negative nitrogen balance	Gontzea et al.[30]
Bicycle ergometer (after 20 days of training)	1.0	55	Zero nitrogen balance	Gontzea et al.[30]

From Dohm GL: Protein nutrition for the athlete. In Hecker AL (ed): Nutritional Aspects of Exercise. Clin Sports Med 3:595, 1984.

Role of Fat During Training

Although fat is a valuable metabolic fuel for muscle activity, high dietary fat intakes do not improve performance.[6] Endurance training significantly increases the ability of muscle to utilize fat. During low-intensity activity, fat may serve as a significant source of energy. The relationship of energy source to the type and length of activity is illustrated in Figure 3–12.[24] Note that even during low-intensity exercise, fats do not represent much over 40 per cent of the fuel supply. The utilization of fat as fuel can only occur under aerobic conditions (with adequate oxygen supply). Additionally, 20 to 30 minutes of exercise are required before blood free fatty acid levels reach concentrations that can help fuel exercise.[3]

Most people have more than 50,000 calories stored in fat. Consequently, low-fat diets will not limit the availability of fat for use as an energy substrate. Even though fats represent an effective energy source for exercise, a high-fat diet does not improve performance. As a matter of fact, high-fat diets may even reduce endurance capacity.[6] This relationship, shown in Figures 3–2 and 3–3, demonstrates that high-fat (low-carbohydrate) diets do not offer the athlete any advantage. Not only do high-fat diets compromise performance, but also these diets may contribute to long-term health problems, such as cardiovascular disease.[46]

Role of Vitamins and Minerals During Training

Vitamins. Vitamins are taken more often than any other nutrient by athletes in search of better performance and health. These vitamins are

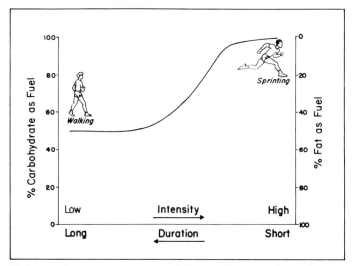

Figure 3–12. As exercise intensity increases and duration decreases, the predominant food fuel shifts toward carbohydrate. (From Fox EL: Sports Physiology. Philadelphia, W.B. Saunders Company, 1979.)

taken even though no scientifically controlled study has ever shown vitamin intake in excess of the RDA to have a beneficial effect on performance.[64]

Most athletes believe that taking large doses (greater than 10 times the RDA) of vitamins is not harmful. This is not true. The fat-soluble vitamins A, D, E, and K can be toxic when taken in high doses.[33] This toxicity (especially for vitamins A and D) results from excess storage of the vitamin in the body. The water-soluble vitamins are not stored in the body; consequently, intakes greater than body requirements are generally excreted through the urine. However, complications such as liver damage, nausea, inflammation of the oral cavity, dermatosis, muscle weakness, and fatigue have been reported for vitamin C, niacin, vitamin B_6, folic acid, and vitamin B_{12} when taken in massive doses on a daily basis.[33]

The use of a daily multivitamin supplement is generally considered safe and may be of some benefit if an athlete has unusual dietary habits or is on a weight-loss program. The exotic dietary habits practiced by some athletes can sometimes precipitate marginal dietary deficiencies. A dietary history can be helpful in identifying these individuals.

Minerals and Electrolytes. A balanced diet is a safe and adequate source of minerals. In general, supplementation with minerals does not enhance physical performance, particularly since exercise does not appear to cause a significant increase in mineral requirements. The possible exception is iron.[56] Female athletes experiencing heavy menstrual blood losses may wish to supplement their diets with extra iron. The iron status of men may also be marginal. Overdoses of iron can be toxic; therefore, individuals who wish to take iron supplements should first consult a physician.

Some individuals advocate the aggressive use of salt tablets. In most cases, salt tablets compound dehydration by accelerating loss of water. Therefore, even when an athlete is sweating excessively (is losing more than 3 to 4 per cent of body weight during the course of a workout on a repeated basis), salt tablets are not necessary and can actually be dangerous.

During some prolonged, intense physical activities, an athlete may experience daily water losses in excess of 5 to 6 per cent of body weight (i.e., pre-season two-a-day football drills, etc.). When individuals are exposed to this amount of body-water loss day after day, an electrolyte deficit may develop.[41] With this degree of dehydration, or during times of heavy sweat loss, some electrolyte replacement should be considered. Electrolytes should be consumed in very dilute solutions during physical activity. A good guideline to follow is the recommendation of the American College of Sports Medicine (ACSM).[2] The ACSM recommends a maximum of 10 mEq (230 mg) of sodium, 10 mEq (355 mg) of chloride, and 5 mEq (195 mg) of potassium per liter of solution. These concentrations are adequate to correct any potential deficit but are not high enough to slow the gastric emptying of the resultant solution or to cause an osmotic overload in the plasma.

PRE-EVENT NUTRITION

The primary goal of the pre-event meal is to provide energy and fluid to support the athlete during competition. Selecting or restricting certain types of foods before competition can prevent or reduce gastrointestinal complications. Most athletes have several foods that cause gastrointestinal distress. These foods differ among athletes, but may include spicy ingredients, gas-producing foods, and high-bulk or high-fat foods. Although high-carbohydrate meals are most appropriate before competition, some athletes have a strong psychological need for certain foods (for example, meat). If so, this perceived need should be accommodated until the athlete understands the benefits of a carbohydrate meal.

New dietary practices should never be instituted on the day of an important competition. The athlete should be given the opportunity to experience any new nutritional program well in advance of competition.

In general, the pre-game meal should have the following characteristics:

1. *High carbohydrate content.* Carbohydrate as 60 to 70 per cent of total calories supports blood glucose levels during competition.

2. *Low fat and low protein content.* Fat slows gastric emptying, and protein can aggravate dehydration.

3. *Low salt content.* High salt levels can cause greater water losses.

4. *Minimal bulk foods.* Bulk foods increase gastrointestinal residue, which in an anxious athlete can lead to vomiting or diarrhea.

5. *Adequate fluid availability.* One or two 8-ounce glasses of water or juice will help ensure adequate hydration.

The pre-game meal must be consumed far enough in advance of the contest to allow for adequate stomach emptying and intestinal digestion. A heavy meal can be consumed three to four hours before competition. In contrast, a light, carbohydrate-based meal can be tolerated when eaten two to three hours before competition. These recommendations may be conservative, because Girandola and associates showed that the consumption of a 1000-calorie liquid or solid meal (55 per cent, 15 per cent, and 30 per cent of total calories as carbohydrate, protein, and fat, respectively) as close as 30 minutes before a maximal run on a treadmill caused no detrimental effects on either metabolic or circulatory parameters.[28] However, this study could not simulate the emotional factors present before and during an athletic contest, and these emotions may be associated with nausea, vomiting, or even diarrhea. Consequently, to be safe, the interval between the pre-event meal and competition should not be any shorter than approximately two hours, even if a small high-carbohydrate solid meal or liquid nutritional supplement is used.

Liquid nutritionals (for example, Ensure) may be beneficial as pre-event feedings. These products are emptied rapidly from the stomach, are easily ingested, and are well-balanced sources of nutrients. Stevens et al. reported approximately 70 per cent of a 500-calorie meal (500 ml) emptied from the stomach within 60 minutes, with almost complete emptying within two hours.[58] These feedings also provide rapid availability of nutrients.[57] This digestibility is reflected in low stool residue, which can be beneficial in the weight-control athlete, such as the wrestler, by minimizing the weight associated with the contents of the gastrointestinal tract.[61] Liquid meals may also be helpful in avoiding the pregame nausea sometimes associated with solid foods.[54]

Liquid meals have been recommended for day-long competitive events, such as swimming and track, and for some tournament situations, such as tennis, basketball, wrestling, and other sports.[45] In these circumstances, the athletes have little time for (or interest in) food. These formulas can also provide a practical solution to the need for supplementation during training to support weight gain or maintenance.[4]

NUTRITIONAL SUPPORT DURING COMPETITION

The impact of nutritional support during competition is dictated by the type of exercise. Short-term, explosive activities such as sprinting will not be limited by nutrition-related factors, assuming that the athlete has a reasonable nutritional status prior to the event. In contrast, performance in long-term events such as distance running and soccer can be influenced by how certain nutrient intakes are managed during the course of the event. This approach applies to practice as well as actual competition. Water and carbohydrates are the only nutrients of concern during practice and competition. The vital importance of water was stressed in the previous discussion of the role of fluids during training. Need for water is no different during competition.

The provision of exogenous carbohydrate during activity can be beneficial, particularly for high-intensity, long-term work bouts. The limited store of muscle and liver glycogen often cannot meet the demands of the exercise. Also, glycogen is not synthesized during activity. If muscle glycogen becomes depleted, the only other source of glucose is the blood. Wahren found that blood glucose may supply as much as 35 to 40 per cent of total energy of exercising muscle.[62] The increased utilization causes a concurrent drop in arterial levels of glucose (Fig. 3–13). Therefore, if glucose declines from the normal blood content of approximately 90 mg/dl to 50 or 40 mg/dl, the exercising muscle fibers cannot obtain enough glucose from the blood and must look elsewhere for fuel. As a result, more muscle glycogen is metabolized, causing it to be used up more rapidly. These interrelationships suggest that the maintenance of a "normal" blood glucose level is beneficial in delaying the onset of muscle fatigue, particularly during long-term work bouts.

Bergstrom and Hultman found that glucose infusions could delay muscle glycogen depletion by 24 per cent during a 60-minute bicycle exercise bout.[7] Several investigations in humans using different work intensities have indicated that the provision of exogenous carbohydrate

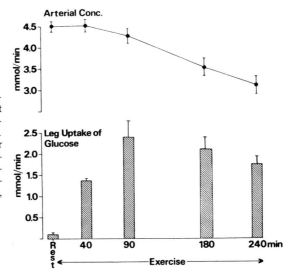

Figure 3–13. Arterial concentration and leg uptake of glucose at rest and during 4 hours of prolonged exercise (mean ± SE). (From Wahren J: Glucose turnover during exercise in man. In The Marathon: Physiological, Medical, Epidemiology and Psychological Studies. Ann NY Acad Sci 301:45, 1977.)

during the exercise period delays the onset of fatigue.[11, 19, 37, 38, 43] The work loads ranged from 45 to 85 per cent of $\dot{V}O_2$ max for periods up to five hours in duration. Figure 3–14 describes the results of one of these trials.[43] The carbohydrate solution prolonged treadmill running by 46.3 and 24.1 minutes compared with no fluid or water replacement, respectively.

Although the mode of action is unclear, the consensus is that the beneficial effect of exogenous carbohydrate is related to the preservation of muscle and liver glycogen.

ENERGY DRINKS

The practical aspects of supplementing an athlete with carbohydrate during competition have not been completely resolved. In general, if an energy drink is to be prepared, the carbohydrate chosen must permit the delivery of a maximal concentration of carbohydrate without compromising the hydration characteristics of the solution, because water must remain the first priority of any such solution.

A fluid-energy replacement beverage should have the following characteristics:

1. *Provide a rapidly available source of water.* The beverage must empty from the stomach as quickly as plain water.
2. *Deliver a significant quantity of easily digested and absorbed carbohydrate.*
3. *Provide an appropriate concentration of important minerals and electrolytes.*
4. *Possess "refreshing" taste characteristics.*

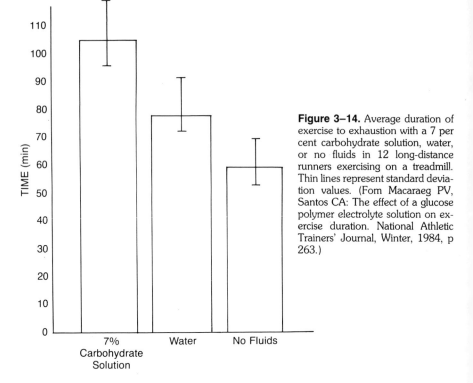

Figure 3–14. Average duration of exercise to exhaustion with a 7 per cent carbohydrate solution, water, or no fluids in 12 long-distance runners exercising on a treadmill. Thin lines represent standard deviation values. (Fom Macaraeg PV, Santos CA: The effect of a glucose polymer electrolyte solution on exercise duration. National Athletic Trainers' Journal, Winter, 1984, p 263.)

Any fluid-energy replacement beverage should be consumed (1) cold (40° to 50°F); (2) in relatively small quantities (start with 100 to 300 ml and adjust to individual preference); and (3) at frequent intervals (every 15 to 20 minutes).

Exercise *does not* necessarily compromise gastrointestinal function. Two studies have shown that stomach emptying time and intestinal absorption are not significantly reduced even at exercise intensities exceeding 75 per cent of $\dot{V}O_2$max.[17, 22] Of course, at intensities above that, fatigue will result quickly for reasons unrelated to fluid availability from the gastrointestinal tract.

Since water delivery is critical, other ingredients in a fluid-energy replacement beverage should not slow the rate of gastric emptying. Carbohydrates and electrolytes have been associated with delayed gastric emptying when fed in high concentrations. Glucose or sucrose cannot be fed at levels exceeding 2.5 per cent without significantly slowing gastric emptying.[17] However, this concentration is too low to have a significant effect on energy needs. The work of Foster indicates that glucose polymers (Polycose Glucose Polymers) could be fed in higher concentrations than glucose without slowing stomach emptying.[23] Studies by Seiple et al.,[55] Macaraeg and Santos,[43] and Norris et al.[48] suggest that a combination of glucose polymers and fructose (5 per cent and 2 per cent, respectively)

TABLE 3–5. Volume of Fluid (ml) Emptied from Stomach*

Subject	30 Min			60 Min		
	H_2O	5% CHO†	7% CHO†	H_2O	5% CHO†	7% CHO†
1	350.8	370.4	339.6	395.7	397.7	378.9
2	372.8	389.2	386.3	395.3	400.0	400.0
3	400.0	342.2	342.3	395.6	384.6	379.4
4	355.4	308.3	355.6	362.5	335.5	382.1
5	388.3	388.8	365.3	396.8	391.7	393.7
6	400.0	359.8	359.7	400.0	399.1	389.9
Mean	377.9	359.8	358.1	391.0	384.8	387.3
SE	3.61	5.15	2.84	2.34	4.14	1.43

*After ingestion of 400 ml of water or carbohydrate solution. Values corrected for gastric secretion.
†Polymerized glucose/fructose-electrolyte solution.
From Seiple RS, Vivian VM, Fox EL, et al: Gastric emptying characteristics of two glucose polymer-electrolyte solutions. Med Sci Sports Exerc 15:366, 1983.

can be used to meet the criteria for a fluid-energy replacement beverage. They reported both a gastric emptying time equivalent to that of water and improved performance (Fig. 3–14, Table 3–5).

The timing of carbohydrate consumption before and during exercise is important. If improperly coordinated, work capability will be compromised. Figure 3–15 describes the effect of a 70-gram pre-exercise sugar load on blood glucose levels and work performance.[15] The elevated blood glucose level increases insulin output, which in turn suppresses mobilization of free fatty acids from the adipose tissue and lowers the liver's ability to release glucose. The net result can be the early onset of hypoglycemia and a premature utilization of muscle glycogen stores, leading to decreased performance capacity. However, Lamb and associates, using the same type of protocol, fed a similar sugar load only five minutes before exercise and found no evidence of an insulin backlash.[40]

Of course, if carbohydrate is consumed earlier than one hour before exercise, there will be adequate time for the glucose-insulin interaction to return to normal, thus eliminating any chance of an insulin backlash.

Levine et al. have reported that fructose does not precipitate this response and thus is preferred to glucose.[42] Fructose, when fed 30 minutes before exercise, maintained stable blood glucose and insulin levels and did not compromise work capacity. In contrast, Fruth and Gisolfi found that fructose, when fed after the onset of exercise, had no demonstrable advantage over glucose.[27] In fact, the consumption of 120 grams of fructose over a two-hour period precipitated complaints of gastrointestinal distress in the subjects. Presumably the presence of glucose would help alleviate this problem since it is an actively absorbed sugar and would stimulate the uptake of the facilitatively absorbed fructose. This combination was used by Seiple et al.,[55] Macaraeg and Santos,[43] and Norris et al.[48] without any problem. The specific role of fructose in exercise has not been resolved and requires further investigation.

Soda loading—the ingestion of sodium bicarbonate to neutralize the buildup of lactic acid in muscles during exercise—has been practiced by

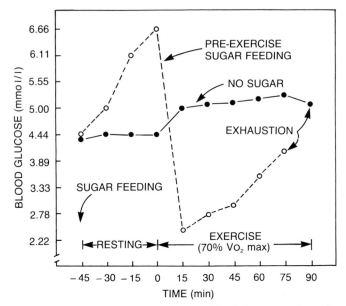

Figure 3–15. Effects of pre-exercise CHO feedings on blood glucose, insulin, and work time to exhaustion. (From Costill DL, Miller JM: Nutrition for endurance sport: Carbohydrate and fluid balance. Int J Sports Med 1:7, 1980.)

many athletes. Work by several investigators has indicated that under high-intensity exercise conditions (i.e., 800-meter or 1500-meter dashes), there is a beneficial effect associated with the consumption of approximately 300 mg/kg body weight of sodium bicarbonate.[29, 49, 63] Even though these preliminary findings suggest that soda loading can help performance, there are several other critical issues that should be considered before attempting to use the material.[18] Severe gastrointestinal distress (diarrhea) has been observed. Half of Gledhill's subjects experienced diarrhea within a half hour of consuming the bicarbonate.[29] Furthermore, because of the high sodium content there may be increased water retention and for some individuals increased hypertension. Additionally, the ethical aspect of this practice is in question. At present, soda loading must be considered a "doping" agent and should not be part of a legitimate sports program.

POST-EVENT NUTRITION

Once competition has been completed for the day, nutritional management is no different than it is during training. Since it is important for the individual to recover from the stress of competition and to return to normal training, efforts should be made to restore body energy and fluid reserves as quickly as possible. Athletes involved in multiple event competition, such as swimming meets, track meets, or wrestling tournaments, represent a special problem. When compounded with a degree of competitive anxiety, these circumstances are often not compatible with solid food consumption. Since the amount of time between events varies from a few minutes to several hours, one nutritional plan cannot fit every situation.

High-intensity exercise, for most people, tends to suppress appetite. Therefore, it is unrealistic to expect athletes to be "hungry" immediately following competition or a strenuous training bout. However, liquid feedings usually can be consumed without problems. These solutions should be prepared as carbohydrate-containing feedings to ensure a rapid availability of blood glucose to maximize glycogen resynthesis. Fox et al. suggest that nutritionally complete liquid diets can be used to meet these needs.[26] (See section on pre-event nutrition for additional information on liquid nutritionals.) Regardless, every attempt should be made to consume a high carbohydrate meal as soon as schedules and appetite permit.

WEIGHT CONTROL

Weight-control sports such as wrestling and light-weight crew present a special nutritional problem. Athletes in these sports must simultaneously be well nourished and hydrated while attaining a minimal body weight. Too often these individuals have unacceptable weight-control practices that can be dangerous to their health. Diuretics, intermittent starvation, excessive sweating via saunas or plastic sweatsuits, induced vomiting, and laxatives are all used by athletes trying to lose weight. The food restriction, fluid deprivation, and dehydration associated with these practices cause reduced muscle strength and stamina and impair thermoregulatory processes.[34] As pointed out earlier, these problems cannot be overcome by eating and drinking during the period between weigh-in and competition. Some sports physicians believe that some weight-control practices used by adolescents can result in growth arrest leading to a reduced mature body size.[32]

Many of the problems caused by rapid weight reduction can be avoided by initiating a weight-control program well in advance of the competitive season. Weight-control should start one to two months before competition, depending on the desired weight loss. This long lead time eliminates dangerous "crash dieting." Athletes in weight-control sports should have body fat determined (via skinfold or underwater weighing) before the diet is started. A reasonable competitive weight then should be projected, taking into account that these individuals will also grow during the season. A series of skinfold thickness categories that can be used to estimate total body fat are described in Table 3–6.[10, 24, 31]

Several guidelines should be kept in mind when planning weight-control programs:

Weight Gain

1. One pound of muscle is equivalent to approximately 2500 Calories; therefore, if an individual is to gain a pound of muscle mass in one

TABLE 3–6. Classification of Body Fat from Skinfold Thickness for Male and Female Athletes*

Classification	Body Fat	Skinfold Thickness (mm)			
		TRICEPS	SCAPULAR	ABDOMEN	SUM
Male					
Lean	<7%	<7	<8	<10	<25
Acceptable	7–15%	7–13	8–15	10–20	25–48
Overfat	>15%	>13	>15	>20	>48
Female					
Lean	<12%	<9	<7	<7	<23
Acceptable	12–25%	9–17	7–14	7–15	23–46
Overfat	>25%	>17	>14	>15	>46

*From Fox EL: Sports Physiology. Philadelphia, W. B. Saunders Company, 1979.

week, he or she must exceed normal requirements by that amount. A balanced nutritional regimen should be used.

2. A weight gain of more than one to one and one-half pounds per week should not be attempted. The athlete should not consume more than 1000 Calories per day in excess of normal required intake. Excessive calories will promote fat deposition.

3. A vigorous exercise program must be employed simultaneously with increased nutrient intake. An increased food intake without an appropriate training program results in increased body fat.

Weight Loss

1. One pound of fat is equivalent to approximately 3500 Calories; consequently, a deficit of 3500 Calories is required to lose one pound of fat.

2. The rate of loss should not exceed approximately two pounds per week. Rates faster than this may be dangerous, particularly in young boys and girls.

3. Dietary intake should not fall below 2000 Calories per day for young boys and 1700 Calories per day for girls. Fewer calories may compromise growth, particularly if the boys and girls are involved in a vigorous training program. Restrictions greater than the above, even in adults, will compromise performance.

4. A specific training program should be combined with dietary restrictions to promote fat loss while preserving lean body mass. If the muscles aren't stimulated to maintain their mass, reduced food intake alone will result in some loss of protein along with the fat.

SUMMARY

Although it is widely accepted that a poor nutritional state is incompatible with optimal physical performance, proper dietary guidelines are not always followed. Too often nutrition is considered as the last resort—and then primarily as some form of witchcraft. Sound nutritional practices should be applied on a daily basis, not just a few hours before competition. The nutritional regimen for an athlete should be designed around four critical nutrition periods:

1. NUTRITIONAL MAINTENANCE DURING TRAINING

—Monitor hydration status carefully because moderate fluid deficits (i.e., 2 to 3 per cent of body weight) can limit endurance, power and cognitive ability. During repetitive, high-fluid loss exercise bouts, thirst cannot be relied on to maintain satisfactory hydration status.

—The diet should contain increased quantities of carbohydrate (i.e., 60 to 70 per cent of total caloric intake) to ensure that chronic glycogen depletion doesn't occur. The form of the carbohydrate (either complex starches or simple sugars) and the number of meals per day are not critical.

—Excessive intakes of protein, vitamins, or minerals are not related to improved performance. It is not necessary for daily protein consumption to exceed 1.5 grams per kilogram of body weight. Both fat- and water-soluble vitamins can cause toxic side effects when consumed in mega doses (10 times the Recommended Dietary Allowance). Normal self-selected diets may be deficient in iron, so athletes, especially females, should be monitored for iron status.

—Athletes experiencing repetitive prolonged work bouts (two-a-day drills) in hot humid environments may need additional mineral intake (i.e., Na, K, Cl, Mg, and Ca). the recommendations of the American College of Sports Medicine[2] should be followed in formulating a beverage to meet these needs.

—Fat intake should be minimized (less than 30 per cent of total calories) since there is no beneficial effect, and in some individuals there may be long-term health concerns.

2. PRE-EVENT NUTRITION

—The provision of fluid and energy should be the primary goal of the pre-competition meal.

—Carbohydrate and fluid intake should be emphasized.

—Foods high in fat, protein, salt, or bulk should be avoided since they could compromise performance by causing gastrointestinal problems or by aggravating dehydration.

3. NUTRITIONAL SUPPORT DURING COMPETITION/TRAINING

—Water and carbohydrate are the main nutrients of concern during practice and competition. Carbohydrate intake during exercise can be beneficial, particularly for high-intensity, long-term work bouts.

—Carbohydrate form and concentration are important. Glucose and sucrose are not considered effective carbohydrates for hydration-energy drinks because at concentrations exceeding 2.5 per cent they slow gastric emptying, thus minimizing energy availability and reducing fluid delivery. Glucose polymers appear to be more effective since they do not retard gastric emptying even at higher concentrations (i.e., 7 per cent).

—Electrolyte intake is usually of minimal concern unless the athlete is unacclimatized and working under hot, humid conditions. These circumstances may contribute to a net negative mineral status. This can be avoided by extra use of the salt shaker at meals and by providing small quantities of minerals in an energy-hydration drink. The ACSM guidelines should be followed when formulating such a solution.

4. POST-EVENT NUTRITION

—Fluids and carbohydrate should be made available as soon as the athlete's schedule will permit. This is particularly important if the athlete is involved in multiple event competition or vigorous daily training bouts. Muscle and liver glycogen stores must be replaced rapidly in preparation for the work bout. The avoidance of dehydration and/or chronic glycogen depletion is essential for successful future performance.

Optimal nutrition is a basic training component necessary for the development and maintenance of top physical performance. A good diet in itself cannot provide fitness or championship form, but a poor diet can ruin both.

ACKNOWLEDGMENT: The author wishes to acknowledge the generous assistance of Bea Armstrong for preparing the manuscript, Wendy Bachhuber for her editorial comments, and Dr. Keith Wheeler for his critical review.

REFERENCES

1. Adolph EF, Dill DB: Observations on water metabolism in the desert. Am J Physiol 123:369, 1983.
2. American College of Sports Medicine: Prevention of heat injuries during distance running. Position Statement. Med Sci Sports 7:VIII, 1975.
3. Askew EW: Role of fat metabolism in exercise. In Hecker AL (ed): Nutritional Aspects of Exercise. Clin Sports Med 3:605, 1984.
4. Bartels RL, Porcello LA, Beam WC, et al: Seasonal body composition changes in male college competitive swimmers: A two part study. In Fox E (ed): Nutrient Utilization During Exercise. Columbus, OH, Ross Laboratories, 1983.
5. Bergstrom J, Hultman E: The effect of exercise on muscle glycogen and electrolytes in normals. Scand J Clin Lab Invest 18:16, 1966.
6. Bergstrom J, Hermanson L, Hultman E, et al: Diet, muscle glycogen and physical performance. Acta Physiol Scand 71:140, 1967.
7. Bergstrom J, Hultman E: A study of glycogen metabolism during exercise in man. Scand J Clin Lab Invest 19:218, 1967.
8. Bijlani RL, Sharma KN: Effect of dehydration and a few regimens of rehydration on human performance. Indian J Physiol Pharmacol 24:255, 1980.

9. Buskirk E, Impietro P, Bass D: Work performance and dehydration effects of physical condition and heat acclimatization. J Appl Physiol 12:189, 1958.
10. Buskirk E: Nutrition for the athlete. In Ryan A, Allman F (eds): Sports Medicine. New York, Academic Press, 1974.
11. Christensen EH, Hanson O: Hypoglhamie, arbeitsfähigkeit und ernäkrung. Scand Arch Physiol 81:172, 1939.
12. Claremont A, Costill DL, Fink WJ, et al: Heat tolerance following diuretic induced dehydration. Med Sci Sports 8:239, 1976.
13. Cohen P, Himms HG, Provel CG: How does insulin stimulate glycogen synthesis? Biochem Soc Symp 43:69, 1979.
14. Consolazio CF, Johnson HL, Nelson RA, et al: Protein metabolism during intensive physical training in the young adult. Am J Clin Nutr 28:29, 1975.
15. Costill DL, Miller JM: Nutrition for endurance sport: Carbohydrate and fluid balance. Int J Sports Med 1:2, 1980.
16. Costill DL, Sherman WM, Fink WJ, et al: The role of dietary carbohydrates in muscle glycogen resynthesis after strenuous running. Am J Clin Nutr 34:1831, 1981.
17. Costill DL, Saltin B: Factors limiting gastric emptying during rest and exercise. J Appl Physiol 37:679, 1974.
18. Costill DL: "Acid-base" balance during repeated bouts of exercise: Influence of HCO_3. Int J Sports Med 5:228, 1984.
19. Coyle EF: Effects of glucose polymers feeding on fatigability and the metabolic response to prolonged exercise. In Fox EL (ed): Nutrient Utilization During Exercise. Columbus, OH, Ross Laboratories, 1983.
20. Dill DB: Life, Heat and Altitude: Physical Effects of Hot Climates and Great Heights. Cambridge, Harvard University Press, 1938.
21. Dohm GL: Protein nutrition for the athlete. In Hecker AL (ed): Nutritional Aspects of Exercise. Clin Sports Med 3:595, 1984.
22. Fordtran JS, Saltin B: Gastric emptying and intestinal absorption during prolonged severe exercise. J Appl Physiol 23:331, 1967.
23. Foster C: Gastric emptying characteristics of glucose polymers. In Fox EL (ed): Nutrient Utilization During Exercise, Columbus, OH, Ross Laboratories, 1983.
24. Fox EL: Sports Physiology. Philadelphia, W. B. Saunders Company, 1979.
25. Fox EL, Mathews DK: The Physiological Basis of Physical Education and Athletics, 3rd ed. Philadelphia, Saunders College Press, 1981.
26. Fox EL, Keller J, Bartels RJ, et al: Multiple daily exercise: Solid vs liquid diets (Abstract). Med Sci Sports 11:102, 1979.
27. Fruth JM, Gisolfi CV: Effects of carbohydrate consumption on endurance performance: Fructose versus glucose. In Fox EL (ed): Nutrient Utilization During Exercise, Columbus, OH, Ross Laboratories, 1983.
28. Girandola RN, Wiswell RA, Frisch F, et al: Effects of liquid and solid meals and time of feeding on VO_2 max. In Fox EL (ed): Nutrient Utilization During Exercise, Columbus, OH, Ross Laboratories, 1983.
29. Gledhill, N: Bicarbonate ingestion and anaerobic performance. Sports Med 1:177, 1984.
30. Gontzea I, Sutzescu R, Dumitrache S: The influence of adaptation to physical effort on nitrogen balance in man. Nutr Rep Int 11:231, 1975.
31. Hill L: Anthropometric estimations of body density of women athletes in selected athletic activities, Dissertation. The Ohio State University, Columbus, OH, 1977.
32. Hansen N: Wrestling with making weight. Phys Sport Med 6:107, 1978.
33. Herbert V: Nutrition Cultism: Facts and Fiction. Philadelphia, G. F. Stickley Company, 1980.
34. Hodges RE, Krehl WA: The role of carbohydrates in lipid metabolism. Am J Clin Nutr 17:334, 1965.
35. Houston ME, Marrin DA, Green HJ et al: The effect of rapid weight loss on physiological functions in wrestlers. Phys Sports Med 9:73, 1981.
36. Hultman E, Nilsson LH: Liver glycogen in man: Effect of diet and exercise. In Pernow P, Saltin B (eds): Muscle metabolism during exercise. New York, Plenum Press, 1971.
37. Ivy JL, Costill DL, Fink WJ, et al: Influence of caffeine and carbohydrate feedings on endurance performance. Med Sci Sports, 11:6, 1979.

38. Ivy JL, Miller VD, Goodyear LG, et al: Endurance improved by ingestion of a glucose polymer supplement. Med Sci Sports Exerc 15:466, 1983.
39. Iyengar A, Nageswara Rao BS: Effect of varying energy and protein intake on nitrogen balance in adults engaged in heavy manual labor. Br J Nutr 41:19, 1979.
40. Lamb DR, Baur T, Connors D, et al: Maltodextrin feeding immediately before prolonged cycling at 62% $\dot{V}_{O_2}$ max increase time to exhaustion (Abstract). Med Sci Sports Exerc 15:126, 1983.
41. Lane HW, Roessler GS, Nelson EW, et al: Effect of physical activity on human potassium metabolism in a hot humid environment. Am J Clin Nutr 31:838, 1978.
42. Levine L, Evans WJ, Cadarette BS, et al: Fructose and glucose ingestion and muscle glycogen use during submaximal exercise. J Appl Physiol 55:1767, 1983.
43. Macaraeg PVJ, Santos CA: The effect of glucose polymer-electrolyte solutions on exercise duration. Proc Aust Sports Med Fed 8:29, 1984.
44. Marable NL, Hickson JF, Korslund MK, et al: Urinary nitrogen excretion as influenced by a muscle-building exercise program and protein intake level. Nutr Rep Int 19:795, 1979.
45. McArdle WD, Katch FI, Katch VL: Exercise physiology: Energy, nutrition and human performance. Philadelphia, Lea and Febiger, 1981.
46. McGill HC, Mott GE: Diet and coronary heart disease. Nutr Rev 4:376, 1976.
47. Merkim G, Spring S: Carbohydrate loading: A dangerous practice. JAMA 223:1511, 1973.
48. Norris WA, Fox EL, Bartels RJ, et al: Rehydration using a glucose polymer-fructose electrolyte solution following prolonged heavy exercise (Abstract). Med Sci Sports Exerc 14:117, 1982.
49. Pate RR, Smith PE, Lambert MJ, et al: Effect of orally administered sodium bicarbonate on performance of high intensity exercise (Abstract). Med Sci Sports Exerc 17:200, 1985.
50. Pitts G, Johnson HL, Consolazio CF: Work in the heat as affected by intake of water, salt and glucose. Am J Physiol 142:253, 1944.
51. Recommended Dietary Allowances, 9th ed. Washington, DC, National Academy of Sciences, 1980.
52. Robinson S, Sadowski B, Newton JL: The effects of dehydration on the aerobic and anaerobic capacities of men. NASA Accession No. N 67–28008. NSG 408. Final Scientific Report, part IV, 1966.
53. Robinson S: The effects of dehydration on performance. In Football Injuries. Washington, DC, National Academy of Sciences, 1970.
54. Rose KD, Schneider PJ, Sullivan GF: A liquid pre-game meal for athletes. JAMA 178:30, 1961.
55. Seiple RS, Vivian VM, Fox EL, et al: Gastric emptying characteristics of two glucose polymer-electrolyte solutions. Med Sci Sports Exerc 15:366, 1983.
56. Smith NJ: Food for Sport. Palto Alto, CA, Bull Publishing Company, 1976.
57. Steinbaugh ML: Nutrient digestibility of complete nutritional liquid diets. In Fox EL (ed): Nutrition Utilization During Exercise. Columbus, OH, Ross Laboratories, 1983.
58. Stevens C, Costill DL, Maxwell B: Impact of carbohydrate source and osmolality on gastric emptying rates of liquid nutritionals (Abstract). J Parent Ent Nutr 3:3, 1979.
59. Torranin C, Smith DP, Byrd RJ: The effect of acute thermal dehydration and rapid rehydration on isometric and isotonic endurance. J Sports Med 19:1, 1979.
60. Torun B, Scrimshaw NS, Young VR: Effect of isometric exercise on body potassium and dietary protein requirements of young men. Am J Clin Nutr 30:1983, 1977.
61. Vivian VM, Snook JT, Hecker AL: Stool characteristics resulting from defined formula diets (Abstract). J Parent Ent Nutr 5:570, 1981.
62. Wahren J: Glucose turnover during exercise in man. In The Marathon: Physiological, Medical, Epidemiology and Psychological Studies. Ann NY Acad Sci 301:45, 1977.
63. Wilkes D, Gledhill N, Smyth R: Effect of acute induced metabolic alkalosis on 800-m racing time. Med Sci Sports Exerc 15:277, 1983.
64. Williams M: Nutritional Aspects of Human Physical and Athletic Performance. Springfield, IL, Charles C Thomas, 1976.
65. Young C, Hutlker L, Scanlon S, et al: Metabolic effects of meal frequency on normal young men. J Am Diet Assoc 61:391, 1972.

4

BLOOD DOPING, OXYGEN BREATHING, AND ALTITUDE TRAINING

BJÖRN EKBLOM, M.D.

PHYSIOLOGICAL BACKGROUND

In sports, many factors influence performance. The physiological factors can be grouped into three areas: energy liberation, neuromuscular function, and mental-psychological function. In this chapter, only the aerobic (oxygen-requiring) energy yield in exercise will be discussed.

In events in which large muscle groups are used, such as cross-country skiing or uphill running, successful athletes have high maximal aerobic power. (This alone does not guarantee good performance.) Maximal aerobic power may be limited at many points in the oxygen transport system. However, most exercise physiologists now agree that factors related to the central circulation limit maximal aerobic power. These factors are the maximal cardiac output and arterial oxygen content. Cardiac output is equal to heart rate times stroke volume. Arterial oxygen content is equal to the hemoglobin concentration times the saturation of hemoglobin by oxygen, plus a small amount of oxygen dissolved in plasma.

Not all of the oxygen offered by the central circulation is used by the muscles. That depends on how much blood is distributed to the muscles and how efficiently they extract oxygen from capillary blood. Maximal oxygen consumption by all tissues of the body is equal to the maximal oxygen uptake of the lungs ($\dot{V}O_2max$). This value, in turn, is

53

equal to the maximal cardiac output ($\dot{Q}_{max}$) times the difference between arterial and mixed venous oxygen content [(a-v)O_{2diff}]:

$$\dot{V}O_{2max} = \dot{Q}_{max} \times (a\text{-}v)O_{2diff}$$

Maximal aerobic power appears to be the most important factor determining the speed that an individual can maintain during the first 10 to 20 minutes of a long-distance event. However, endurance—how long the individual can continue to exercise at that speed—is determined largely by local muscle factors such as enzyme activities, glycogen content, muscle fiber distribution, and capillary density. Thus, both central and local factors are important in aerobic exercise.

This chapter deals with the problems of how maximal aerobic power and aerobic performance are modified if the arterial oxygen content is changed by one of the following methods: (1) changes in hemoglobin concentration, including "blood doping," (2) oxygen breathing, and (3) training at altitude. No attempt has been made in this chapter to evaluate effects on nonaerobic events, which rely mainly on anaerobic capacity, muscle strength, and coordination.

CHANGES IN HEMOGLOBIN CONCENTRATION (BLOOD DOPING)

When arterial oxygen content is lowered, maximal aerobic power is reduced. Arterial oxygen content decreases following blood loss, upon exposure to hypoxia (low oxygen) at high altitude, and when some of the hemoglobin is blocked by carbon monoxide poisoning. During maximal exercise, the body cannot compensate further for the lower arterial oxygen content because cardiac output can go no higher. In addition, no more oxygen can be extracted from capillary blood because most of it already has been used by the exercising muscle.

Conversely, could maximal aerobic power be increased by increasing hemoglobin concentration and, consequently, arterial oxygen content? There are several reasons to think that this might not be the case. Increased blood viscosity might cause a decrease in maximal cardiac output. Also, skeletal muscle might not be able to use the extra oxygen offered to it. Would the muscle enzyme systems be able to use more substrates if more oxygen were available?

In 1966, the first studies addressing these questions were performed in our laboratories. Since that time, five studies have been carried out by us and many more by others. Well-trained subjects were used because, otherwise, the repeated maximal exercise tests would increase their maximal aerobic power and confuse the results.

The basic experimental design for most of these studies was as follows. First, baseline values were obtained for physiological and hematological parameters and for physical performance (running on a treadmill). Then, 800 to 1200 ml of whole blood were withdrawn and stored in a blood bank. (Alternatively, the red cells can be separated and

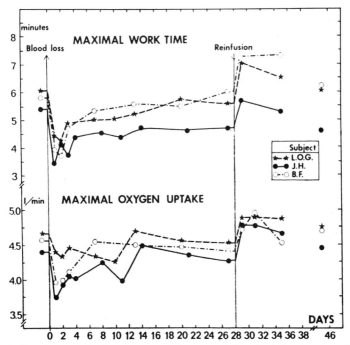

Figure 4–1. Changes in physical performance following withdrawal of blood and reinfusion four weeks later.

frozen for longer periods of time.) The subjects' hemoglobin concentration fell as expected, as did aerobic power and physical performance (Fig. 4–1).

During the four to five weeks after blood was withdrawn, hemoglobin concentration returned to normal. Maximal aerobic power and physical performance also returned to normal in most subjects. At that point, the red blood cells were reinfused. Tests the following days showed that maximal aerobic power increased by an average of about 10 per cent.

In well-trained subjects, an 8 to 10 per cent increase in maximal aerobic power is almost impossible to achieve during a couple of years of hard physical training. In contrast, the differences between top athletes in endurance events is only a fraction of the "overnight" increase in maximal aerobic power described above. Field tests on cross-country runners also showed improved performance following reinfusion of blood. The effects of "blood doping" on maximal aerobic power and physical performance have been confirmed in other laboratories. Regretfully, blood doping also has been used by athletes in competition.

In our studies, enhancement of maximal aerobic power and physical performance lasted from a few days to 18 days after reinfusion of blood. The reason for this variability is not known. Variations also occurred in response to the infusion of a specific red-cell mass, probably because of individual variations in the increase in blood volume. (There was a good correlation between increase in hemoglobin concentration and increase in maximal aerobic power.) Furthermore, it is possible that a given increase in hemoglobin concentration from a low normal value (135 grams per liter) has a greater effect than the same increase from a high normal value (155 grams per liter).

Maximal cardiac output did not change, indicating that the moderate increase in blood viscosity did not impede the central or peripheral circulation. The concentration of 2,3-diphosphoglycerate in red blood cells was unchanged, suggesting that their oxygen-carrying function was not altered. Also, the exercising muscles were able to consume the extra oxygen that was offered to them.

Thus, the theory that increasing the oxygen content of arterial blood can increase maximal aerobic power and improve physical performance is valid. It applies to sports in which large muscle groups are used during prolonged exercise. However, no studies have been reported concerning small muscle groups, mental performance during physical exercise, or performance in team sports.

We experienced no significant adverse effects from blood withdrawal or reinfusion. However, it should be remembered that such procedures can cause medical complications including syncope, hematoma formation, and infection. Competent blood banking techniques are required. All of our subjects received their own blood. If the blood is donated by another individual, additional risks include transfusion reaction and disease transmission.

Reinfusion of blood in sports must be regarded as doping and is unethical. Currently, no method for detecting blood doping is available. Such testing probably would require a sample of venous blood, which is not an acceptable procedure for most competing athletes or sports organizations.

SUMMARY

Increasing arterial oxygen content by increasing the hemoglobin concentration ("blood doping") enhances maximal aerobic power and improves physical performance in endurance sports. This type of manipulation must be regarded as unethical. Presently, there are no methods for the detection of blood doping in sports.

OXYGEN BREATHING

Breathing oxygen *during* exercise increases maximal aerobic power and prolongs time to exhaustion in short-term maximal exercise. During submaximal exercise, breathing oxygen (40 to 60 per cent O_2 in N_2) reduces heart rate and pulmonary ventilation. Such use of oxygen in sports would be regarded as doping.

Breathing oxygen immediately before exercise or during rest periods has been practiced in sports for many years but probably is of little value. The theoretical reason for doing this is to increase arterial oxygen content by increasing both the amount of oxygen dissolved in plasma and the saturation of hemoglobin by oxygen. (Normally, arterial hemoglobin is almost 100 per cent saturated, but this may be reduced somewhat during maximal exercise.) Furthermore, oxygen breathing increases the partial pressure of oxygen in arterial blood, which could be of benefit to the exercising muscle. However, when oxygen breathing is stopped prior to returning to competition, arterial oxygen content returns to normal within a few seconds.

Does breathing oxygen after exercise speed up the elimination of anaerobic metabolites from blood or muscle? There is no evidence that this is so. If such an effect exists, it is very small.

Hyperventilation during and after hard physical exercise is reduced by oxygen breathing. For this reason, the subjective feeling of fatigue and strain on the ventilatory muscles may be reduced, leading to a psychological feeling of faster recovery from exercise. A physiological effect may also exist. Since reduced hyperventilation also reduces the oxygen demand of the respiratory muscles, it might reduce the amount of lactate produced by them.

SUMMARY

Breathing oxygen before exercise has no value. "Sniffing" oxygen in rest periods during prolonged exercise—as in an ice hockey game—may have a psychological effect but has no significant physiological effect.

TRAINING AT HIGH ALTITUDE

At high altitude, the partial pressure of oxygen in inspired air is reduced. For this reason, acute exposure to high altitude reduces arterial oxygen content, which leads to a reduction in maximal aerobic power and endurance. During acclimatization, maximal aerobic power increases gradually but does not return to sea-level values even after several years.

The increase in maximal aerobic power and physical performance that is associated with acclimatization is largely explained by an increase in hemoglobin concentration—somewhat like blood doping. It is also possible that prolonged hypoxia at altitude induces beneficial changes in muscle such as increased capillary density, increased myoglobin concentration, or increased concentrations of enzymes important to aerobic metabolism. All of these factors would improve endurance. Thus, it is reasonable to ask whether training at altitude will enhance physical performance at sea level. Sports experience and scientific data suggest not.

In 1968, the Olympic Games were held in Mexico City at an altitude of about 2000 meters (7300 feet). Many of the world's top athletes trained at high altitude for months beforehand. During the season following the Olympic Games, many of these same athletes competed at sea level. The number of world records set was about average. So, it seems that prolonged training at altitude did not enhance sea-level performance.

Similar conclusions can be drawn from South African track championships that are held alternately at high altitude and sea level. In middle- and long-distance running, athletes who live at altitude have no advantage at sea level. However, they perform better than their low-land competitors when running at high altitude.

Several laboratory investigations have analyzed this problem. Almost all concluded that high altitude training does not enhance sea-level performance. The reason for this is not clear. It appears that the positive effect of increased hemoglobin concentration is counteracted by other factors. The most important factor may be that the intensity of training must be reduced at altitude, resulting in a lower training stimulus. In addition, at extremely high altitudes such as 4000 meters (13,100 feet), the maximal heart rate is decreased. Maximal cardiac output is reduced, but the oxygen content of arterial blood increases with time. Maximal aerobic power and endurance improve with acclimatization but fail to reach sea-level values.

In acute exposure to the hypoxia of altitude, hyperventilation occurs, carbon dioxide is lost, and alkalosis results. In compensation, the kidney excretes bicarbonate ions, and the buffering capacity of blood and tissues decreases. Whether this significantly diminishes tolerance for lactic acid is unknown.

SUMMARY

Sports experience and laboratory studies suggest that training at high altitude does not enhance performance at sea level.

FURTHER READING

Åstrand PO, Rodahl K: Textbook of Work Physiology. New York, McGraw-Hill, 1977.

Buick FJ, Gledhill N, Froese AN, et al: Effect of induced erythrocythemia on aerobic work capacity. J Appl Physiol 48:636, 1980.

Buskirk ER, Kollias J, Akers RF, et al: Maximal performance at altitude and on return from altitude in conditioned runners. J Appl Physiol 23:259, 1967.

Ekblom B, Goldbarg AN, Gullbring B: Response to exercise after blood loss and reinfusion. J Appl Physiol 33:175, 1972.

Ekblom B, Huot R, Stein EM, Thorstensson AT: Effect of changes in arterial oxygen content on circulation and physical performance. J Appl Physiol 39:71, 1975.

Ekblom B, Wilson G, Åstrand PO: Central circulation during exercise after venesection and reinfusion of red blood cells. J Appl Physiol 40:379, 1976.

Goddard RF (ed): The International symposium on the Effects of Altitude on Physical Performance. Chicago, The Altitude Institute, 1967.

Grover J: Performance at altitude. In Strauss RH (ed): Sports Medicine and Physiology. Philadelphia, W. B. Saunders Company, 1979, p 327.

Horstman D, Weiskopf R, Jackson E: Work capacity during 3-wk sojourn at 4,300 m: Effects of relative polycythemia. J Appl Physiol: Respirat Environ Exerc Physiol 49:311, 1980.

Kanstrup IL, Ekblom B: Blood volume and hemoglobin concentration as determinants of maximal aerobic power. Med Sci Sports Exerc 16:256, 1984.

Lambertsen CJ: Effects of oxygen at high partial pressure. In Fenn WO, Rahn H (eds): Handbook of Physiology. Washington, DC, American Physiological Society, 1965, p 1027.

Williams MH, Wesseldine S, Somma T, et al: The effect of induced erythrocythemia upon 5-mile treadmill run time. Med Sci Sports Exerc 13:169, 1981.

5

ANABOLIC STEROIDS

RICHARD H. STRAUSS, M.D.

Anabolic steroids are derivatives of the natural male hormone testosterone (Fig. 5–1). The term "anabolic" means "tissue building." These hormones are also masculinizing, or "androgenic," so their full name is anabolic-androgenic steroid hormones. Their four-ringed steroid structure is also found in corticosteroids such as cortisone. The corticosteroid hormones have anti-inflammatory and other properties that are different from those of the anabolic steroids. Unfortunately, the general public often confuses these two classes of hormones when the word "steroid" is used.

PATTERNS OF USE

Anabolic steroids became available to physicians following World War II and were used in attempts to speed recovery from starvation and major surgery. They have been tried as therapy for osteoporosis, the anemia of renal failure, and alcoholic hepatitis.[1] Currently, anabolic steroids are used therapeutically as replacement for deficient testosterone in males, anemia due to failure of the bone marrow, and hereditary angioneurotic edema.[2] They also are given to transsexual females who wish to be masculinized.

During World War II, anabolic steroids were administered experimentally to increase aggressiveness in German troops.[3] The Russians in 1954 were reportedly the first to use anabolic steroids in an attempt to improve athletic performance,[3] soon to be followed by Americans and others. Initially, these drugs were used in sports requiring great strength or muscle size, such as weight lifting, shot put, and body building. Although the use is still greatest in these sports, athletes from both Eastern and Western blocs have tested positive for anabolic steroids in

59

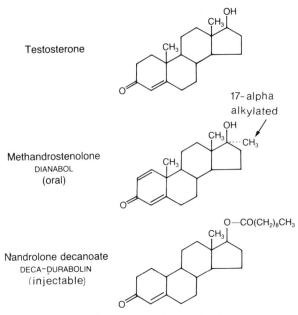

Figure 5–1. Synthetic anabolic-androgenic steroids are related to testosterone in structure and function. (Modified from Strauss RH (ed): Sports Medicine. Philadelphia, W.B. Saunders Company, 1984, p 483.)

sprint and distance running, wrestling, and swimming.[4] Both men and women have been involved. In the United States, anabolic steroids are used by some athletes, including football players, at the professional, college, and high-school levels, and even occasionally by high-school girl runners.

Some of the anabolic steroids used by athletes are listed in Table 5–1. Anabolic steroids are generally used in "cycles"—that is, taken for a period of time, for example eight weeks, then not taken for several weeks or months or taken in lower doses. Up to five types of anabolic steroids may be used simultaneously, a method called "stacking."

MECHANISMS OF ACTION

Anabolic steroids can be taken orally or by injection. The most popular oral anabolic steroid has long been methandrostenolone (Dianabol, Fig. 5–1). Dianabol is no longer manufactured by Ciba, but the generic drug is still made by other companies. One of the most popular injectable preparations in the United States is Deca-Durabolin (Fig. 5–1). Oral anabolic steroids have an alkyl group added at the 17-alpha position to decrease degradation as they pass through the liver following absorption from the intestine.

TABLE 5–1. Anabolic Steroids Used by Two Groups of Athletes[11, 22]

Oral anabolic steroids
Anadrol (oxymetholone)
Anavar (oxandrolone)
Dianabol (methandrostenolone)
Maxibolin (ethylestrenol)
methyltestosterone
Primobolan (methenolone)
Proviron (mesterolone)
Winstrol (stanozolol)

Injectable anabolic steroids
Anatrofin (stenobolone)
Bolfortan (testosterone nicotinate)
Deca-Durabolin (nandrolone decanoate)
Delatestryl (testosterone enanthate)
Depo-Testosterone (testosterone cypionate)
Dianabol (methandrostenolone)
Durabolin (nandrolone phenpropionate)
Enoltestovis (hexoxymestrolum)
Equipoise (boldenone—veterinary)
Primobolan (methenolone enanthate)
Sustanon 250 (a mixture of testosterone esters)
Therobolin
Trophobolene
Wintrol V (stenozolol—veterinary)

Anabolic steroids travel from the bloodstream, through cell walls, into the cytoplasm. Cytoplasmic receptors for testosterone and related male hormones exist in different types of cells and determine the cell's response to anabolic steroids by controlling the production of RNA by DNA.[5] In muscle cells, anabolic steroids have been shown to stimulate the production of muscle protein.[6] Also, anabolic steroids may block the catabolic effect of corticosteroids that are released during stress, thereby decreasing the loss of muscle protein. In addition, both the increased aggression often associated with anabolic steroids and the placebo effect may lead to more strenuous training.

In certain cells, male hormones stimulate secondary sex characteristics such as beard growth and thickening of the vocal cords. Once the cytoplasmic receptors are saturated, higher concentrations of anabolic steroids probably have no further physiological effect. Thus, the huge doses of anabolic steroids currently in use appear to represent overkill.

EFFECTS IN MEN

Do anabolic steroids help to increase muscle size and strength in men? This question has been debated in the scientific literature for many years. The answer now appears to be "yes"—when the individual is experienced in strength training, is performing strenuous strength training concurrently, and is well nourished. For references to the numerous papers both supporting and opposing this conclusion, the reader is referred to the American College of Sports Medicine's Position Stand on "The Use of Anabolic-Androgenic Steroids in Sports," which appears in the appendix of this book. Other reviews[7, 8] also address this question. Although anabolic steroids may help to increase hemoglobin concentration, there is no evidence that they enhance aerobic capacity or endurance.

Do anabolic steroids affect health adversely? The answer is clearly "yes," and it is these side effects that discourage many athletes from using steroids. The use of anabolic steroids results in decreased production of testosterone by the testes. This is thought to occur because the brain's hypothalamus monitors the level of male hormones in the blood and, sensing an excess, decreases the stimulus (gonadotropin-releasing hormone) to the pituitary. The pituitary then releases less luteinizing hormone (LH) and the testes produce less testosterone. Also, less follicle-stimulating hormone (FSH) is released by the pituitary and sperm production falls.[9] For this reason, anabolic-androgenic steroids have been suggested as a male contraceptive[10] but are not reliable as such. A decrease in the size and firmness of the testes is observed with extended use of anabolic steroids. These effects appear to be reversible over a number of weeks or months after steroids are stopped, but no one is entirely sure. Abnormal sperm may persist for weeks or months, so men planning to father a child would be wise to avoid anabolic steroids for a number of months beforehand.

The effect of anabolic steroids on sex drive is highly variable. However, a common pattern is that sex drive increases when steroids are begun and may decrease to normal or below normal after several weeks of use.[11] When steroids are stopped, sex drive usually falls below normal for several weeks until the testes resume production of testosterone. Some users notice no change in sex drive at any time, but occasional men have felt that their sex drive never returned to normal after prolonged steroid use.

Human chorionic gonadotropin (HCG) is sometimes used concurrently with anabolic steroids to prevent testicular atrophy or afterwards to promote quicker resumption of testosterone production by the testes.

Gynecomastia develops in a minority of men who use anabolic steroids because of the metabolism of androgens to estrogens. It appears as a small, firm, tender mass of breast tissue under one or both nipples. Rarely, a small amount of clear fluid is secreted. After steroids are stopped, the breast tissue usually becomes softer and less prominent but does not disappear entirely. Some steroid users have taken anti-estrogen compounds such as tamoxifen (Nolvadex) in an attempt to minimize gynecomastia, but it is not clear that this is effective. Occasionally, the breast tissue is removed surgically for cosmetic reasons, but scarring may be visible.

Acne commonly appears or is made worse with steroid use. Loss of scalp hair and balding are accelerated in men who have inherited a tendency for baldness.[12]

Increased aggressiveness and irritability are common with steroid use. Some athletes consider this an advantage because they "attack the weights" more aggressively. However, problems with interpersonal relationships often occur, such as fights with other athletes, girlfriends, strangers, or walls.

An increased frequency of musculotendinous injury is thought by some to occur, perhaps because muscle strength and motivation increase faster than the strength of the associated tendons and connective tissue.

One of the most important questions about anabolic steroids is, "What are the long-term effects?" Unfortunately, the answer is not clear because these drugs have been in use for a relatively short time by a relatively small number of people. In comparison, consider the millions of people who smoked cigarettes over dozens of years before there was sufficient evidence to conclude that "smoking is hazardous to your health." There is, however, sufficient evidence to cause concern about the long-term effects of anabolic steroids in addition to the short-term effects described above.

When anabolic steroids are used, HDL cholesterol ("the good cholesterol") decreases in plasma and low-density lipoproteins sometimes increase,[13] suggesting a greater risk for cardiovascular disease. Myocardial infarctions have occurred in a few young men who had used anabolic steroids for several years. Increased blood pressure also has been observed.

Liver tumors, both benign and malignant, have been linked with the administration of anabolic steroids as therapy for patients with serious diseases such as aplastic anemia.[14] The 17-alpha-alkylated anabolic (oral) steroids, in particular, were implicated. Peliosis hepatis, in which liver tissue dies and is replaced by blood-filled cysts, also was observed.[15]

In healthy young athletes who used steroids,[16, 17] two cases of liver cancer (hepatocellular carcinoma) have been reported. In addition, two deaths have occurred from malignant kidney tumors (Wilms' tumor) in steroid users.[18]

Moderate elevations of the common liver-function tests SGOT and SGPT do not necessarily indicate liver disease in persons who are training with heavy weights. Small amounts of these enzymes are released from the stressed skeletal muscles, resulting in blood levels moderately higher than normal,[11] which may be misinterpreted as reflecting liver damage by anabolic steroids. Other liver-function tests appear to be reliable; that is, muscular exercise does not cause them to be elevated.

The use of shared needles for the injection of anabolic steroids is associated with the transmission of diseases such as hepatitis B and AIDS.[19]

EFFECTS IN WOMEN

Many of the differences in secondary sexual characteristics between men and women are determined by testosterone. Therefore, it is not surprising that women who take anabolic-androgenic steroid hormones gradually develop masculine secondary sexual characteristics. Women athletes who take anabolic steroids do so because they wish to increase their strength or muscle size. Both of these effects may occur when the women train concurrently with weights. In contrast, women who train with weights but do not take steroids can increase their strength significantly without noticeably increasing muscle size.

Side effects of anabolic steroids in women include growth of facial hair, increased body hair, deepening of the voice, and enlargement of the clitoris.[12, 20–22] These effects appear to be permanent. Effects that seem to return to normal after the male hormones are stopped include menstrual cessation or irregularity, increased libido, increased aggressiveness, and acne. Additional long-term risks that were discussed above for men probably also apply to women.

In general, the extent of anabolic steroid use by women athletes is unknown. In a few, the high doses of anabolic steroids are equal to those used by men.[22] In more moderate doses, steroids are used by some women in sports such as running which do not depend on enormous strength. It appears that the majority of women athletes do not wish to experience the masculinizing effects of anabolic steroids and do not use them.

EFFECTS IN BOYS

Teen-age boys often wish to gain strength or weight. For example, a high-school football player may try to gain 20 pounds of muscle over the summer to improve his chance of playing first-string instead of second-string football. The boys who try anabolic steroids during training may, in fact, achieve an increase in strength or weight. This occurs largely because the boy has accelerated his rate of maturation. He has filled out and reached a level of muscularity that may well have occurred anyway, but has occurred sooner. The drawback is that if the boy has not reached his full height, he may stunt his growth. Anabolic steroids tend to close the growth plates at the ends of bones sooner than normal, permanently decreasing further growth.[23] In our society, height is an advantage; most boys do not wish to be shorter than they normally would be.

GROWTH HORMONE

Human growth hormone (HGH, somatotropin) is not a steroid but a polypeptide hormone produced by the pituitary. In the past few years, athletes have injected human growth hormone in an attempt to increase muscular strength. Some users think it is effective and some do not. There are no scientific studies available to evaluate this question. Growth hormone is usually used in conjunction with anabolic steroids, but because there is currently no practical test for it in sports, it is sometimes used in place of anabolic steroids before contests at which drug testing is done.

During childhood, insufficient quantities of growth hormone result in dwarfism, whereas overproduction causes gigantism. Growth hormone continues to be secreted during adult life. Certain pituitary tumors are capable of producing excessive amounts of growth hormone, which over several years result in the acromegalic syndrome in adults. In acromegaly, height does not increase because growth plates are fused, but bones and connective tissue become so thick that victims can no longer wear their rings or shoes. Facial features become coarser, sometimes grotesque, because of overgrowth of the brow of the skull, the jaw, and soft tissues. The heart, lungs, and liver may double in size. Long-standing acromegaly is characterized by muscular weakness and joint laxity. Growth hormone is diabetogenic.

Human growth hormone is scarce because its source is the pituitary glands of cadavers, and it is expensive—several hundred dollars for a three-week supply. Animal growth hormone from beef or pork may be sold in place of human growth hormone. The solution, sold as "rhesus growth hormone," almost certainly contains no such ingredient because rhesus monkeys are extremely scarce and expensive research animals. Nonhuman growth hormone is completely without physiological effect, although there may be risks associated with injecting these proteins into the body. Such injections may induce growth hormone antibody formation, neutralizing endogenous growth hormone.

Athletes have taken arginine or L-dopa in attempts to stimulate the release of growth hormone from their pituitaries, probably achieving a response that is small, brief, and insignificant. Synthetic growth hormone is produced by bacteria, using recombinant DNA techniques. As this material becomes available in large amounts, the market price probably will drop and its use by athletes will increase. The acromegalic syndrome may then become evident.

Parents have been known to ask for growth hormone for a child, to make him or her a taller basketball player or a larger football player and thus increase the child's chances for a college scholarship. The questionable safety and ethics of this such practice make it inadvisable.

CONTROL OF ANABOLIC STEROIDS IN SPORTS

Athletes who use anabolic steroids argue that they should be allowed to do so without restriction because (1) the drugs are effective at improving athletic performance; (2) the negative effects of the drugs are minimal and acceptable to them; and (3) they have the right to control their own bodies.

Opponents of anabolic steroids argue that (1) performance-enhancing drugs are contrary to the nature of sport; (2) the drugs have adverse effects on health; and (3) the use of these drugs by some athletes forces others to use them to remain competitive.

Efforts to control the use of anabolic steroids by making them unavailable to athletes have been unsuccessful. In many countries these drugs can be purchased without prescription, like vitamins. In the United States they are prescription drugs sold with the same restrictions as antibiotics or anti-inflammatories. Most medical organizations feel that the prescription of anabolic steroids to improve athletic performance is unethical, and most physicians refuse to prescribe them for that purpose. Still, a significant portion of users in the United States get their anabolic steroids from physicians. Most anabolic steroids, however, are purchased on the black market and are readily available at gyms or wherever strength athletes congregate. The cost on the black market is often about the same as or less than the price in pharmacies. Many of the anabolic steroids popular in the United States are manufactured in other countries and imported illegally. Knowledge of the adverse effects of anabolic steroids may well be part of the reason that most athletes do not use them. However, for those persons who feel that steroids are critical to their performance, education probably has a negligible effect.

The detection of anabolic steroid use is discussed in Chapter 8. The testing of athletes' urine at a given contest is partially effective at controlling drug use. That is, such testing discourages anabolic steroid use for a period of time before the contest. Athletes generally avoid using oral anabolic steroids for several weeks and injectable oil-based anabolic steroids for several months before an anticipated test. Earlier use of anabolic steroids, such as that by girls who wish to mature with greater muscularity, is undetectable. In some nations, top athletes are subject to unannounced drug testing at any time—a procedure that is controversial with respect to civil liberties but is probably effective at discouraging drug use.

REFERENCES

1. Mendenhall CL, Anderson S, et al: Short-term and long-term survival in patients with alcoholic hepatitis treated with oxandrolone and prednisolone. N Engl J Med 311:1464–1470, 1984.
2. Wilson JD, Griffin JE: The use and misuse of androgens. Metabolism 29:1278–1295, 1980.
3. Wade N: Anabolic steroids: Doctors denounce them, but athletes aren't listening (news). Science 176:1399–1403, 1972.
4. Shuer M: Steroids. Women Sports 4:17–23, 1982.
5. Rogozkin VA: Anabolic steroid metabolism in skeletal muscle. J Steroid Biochem 11:923–926, 1979.
6. Snochowski M, et al: Androgen and glucocorticoid receptors in human skeletal muscle cytosol. J Steroid Biochem 14:765–771, 1981.
7. Haupt HA, Rovere GD: Anabolic steroids: A review of the literature. Am J Sports Med 12:469–484, 1984.
8. Wright JE: Anabolic steroids and athletics. In Hutton RS, Miller DI (eds): Exerc Sport Sci Rev 8:149–202, 1980.
9. Holma P, Aldercreutz H: Effect of an anabolic steroid (methandienone) on plasma LH-FSH and testosterone and on the response to intravenous administration of LRH. Acta Endocrinol 83:856–864, 1976.

10. Holma PK: Effects of an anabolic steroid (methandienone) on spermatogenesis. Contraception 15:151–162, 1977.
11. Strauss RH, Wright JE, Finerman GAM, et al: Side effects of anabolic steroids in weight-trained men. Phys Sportsmed 11:87–95, 1983.
12. Houssay AB: Effects of anabolic-androgenic steroids on the skin, including hair and sebaceous glands. In Kochakian CD (ed): Anabolic-Androgenic Steroids. New York, Springer-Verlag, 1976.
13. Webb OL, Laskarzewski PM, Glueck CJ: Severe depression of high-density lipoprotein cholesterol levels in weight lifters and body builders by self-administered exogenous testosterone and anabolic-androgenic steroids. Metabolism 33:971–975, 1984.
14. Johnson FL: The association of oral androgenic-anabolic steroids and life threatening disease. Med Sci Sports 7:284–286, 1975.
15. Bagheri SA, Boyer JL: Peliosis hepatis associated with androgenic-anabolic steroid therapy. Ann Intern Med 81:610–618, 1974.
16. Overly WL, et al: Androgens and hepatocellular carcinoma in an athlete. Ann Intern Med 100:158–159, 1984.
17. Goldman B: Liver carcinoma in an athlete taking anabolic steroids. J Am Osteopath Assoc 5:25, 1985.
18. Prat J, et al: Wilms' tumor in an adult associated with androgen abuse. JAMA 237:2322, 1977.
19. Sklarek HM, et al: AIDS in a body builder using anabolic steroids. N Engl J Med 311:1701, 1984.
20. Damste PH: Voice change in adult women caused by virilizing agents. J Speech Hear Disord. 32:126–132, 1967.
21. Kruskemper HL: Anabolic Steroids. New York, Academic Press, 1968.
22. Strauss RH, Liggett MT, Lanese RR: Anabolic steroid use and perceived effects in ten weight-trained women athletes. JAMA 253:2871–2873, 1985.
23. Daniel WA Jr, Benett DL: The use of anabolic-androgenic steroids in childhood and adolescence. In Kochakian CD (ed): Anabolic-Androgenic Steroids. New York, Springer-Verlag, 1976.

6

STIMULANTS

JOHN A. LOMBARDO, M.D.

Fatigue is the enemy of performance, be it on the athletic field, in the classroom, at the podium, or in the business arena. Sleep, relaxation, proper diet, and physical conditioning are all preparations that can be made to battle this enemy. Some individuals find themselves losing this battle, and others, simply to gain an edge over their competition, utilize stimulants. Stimulants are readily available in our everyday life and, with a little effort, all varieties can be obtained. Amphetamines, cocaine, caffeine, and nicotine are all stimulants that have been, and still are in some instances, utilized for enhancement of performance or escape from reality.

Performance in athletics is a multifaceted entity that can be affected by many things. Some factors that influence athletic performance include:

1. Genetic composition
2. Level of fitness
   a. Physical conditioning
   b. State of health
   c. Diet
   d. Sleep
   e. Environment
      1. Climate
      2. Altitude
      3. Pollution
3. Skills and techniques
4. Coaching
5. Psyche
   a. Goals
   b. Arena
   c. Opponent
6. Luck

The weight of each of these factors is of course different, but in the very competitive world of professional and high-level amateur athletics, where many of these factors are similar for any two opponents, a small change in any one area may mean the difference between success and failure (if one views success as winning based on score or place). Many of these factors are not in the athlete's control. Genetic composition, arena, opponent, and luck are out of the athlete's hands. However, level of fitness, skills and technique, psyche, and coaching can all be altered by various methods. One method for enhancing performance is the use of ergogenic aids, which are substances that help to generate increased force or endurance in the athletic endeavor and thereby aid performance. Ergogenic aids are sometimes effective and often illegal (against the rules of the various governing bodies of organized sports, e.g., International Olympic Committee [IOC] or National Collegiate Athletic Association [NCAA]). Stimulants are popular as ergogenic aids owing to their ability to mask, delay, or alter the perception of fatigue.

AMPHETAMINES

HISTORY

Amphetamines were first utilized clinically for nasal congestion, narcolepsy, and obesity in the 1930's.[1, 2, 3] Many compounds have been developed and are listed in Table 6–1 with some common street names.[4] The use of amphetamines by athletes has been documented in Mandel's report concerning "The Sunday Syndrome" in professional football. Anecdotes and personal communication report use among athletes in endurance events and games to combat fatigue.[5, 6]

Therapeutic uses of the amphetamines have included:

1. Obesity (anorexiant)—A specific CNS effect of amphetamines is to decrease appetite.
2. Narcolepsy—CNS stimulation by amphetamines prevents the lapses into normal sleep during periods of monotonous activity or inactivity that are the hallmarks of this uncommon disorder.

TABLE 6–1. Commonly Available Amphetamines

Generic Name	Trade Name	Street Name
Racemic amphetamine sulfate	Benzedrine	bennies, peaches
Dextroamphetamine sulfate	Dexedrine	dexies, oranges, orange hearts
Methamphetamine hydrochloride (desoxyephedrine hydrochloride)	Desoxyn Methampex	meth, crystal, whites
Amphetamine complex (amphetamine and d-amphetamine resin)	Biphetamine	black beauties

Adapted from Morgan JP: Clinical pharmacology of amphetamines. In Smith DE (ed): Amphetamine Use, Misuse and Abuse. Proceedings of the National Amphetamine Conference, 1978. Boston, G. K. Hall and Company, 1979, p 3.

3. Minimal brain dysfunction (hyperkinesis)—Amphetamines have a paradoxical calming effect in the child with minimal brain dysfunction. The drugs (more popular recently is methylphenidate [Ritalin]) are an adjunct to other therapeutic, educational, psychological, and sociological interventions.

4. Depression—Studies have shown that the euphoria-producing potential of amphetamines is more consistent than that of morphine and the barbiturates.

5. Others—Amphetamines have also been used for severe menstrual cramps, in psychotic patients (to counteract the sedation of tranquilizers), and in drug withdrawal programs for amphetamine users.

The use of amphetamines in some of these conditions has decreased or ceased and has been replaced by other medications with less potential for abuse.[1-3]

PHARMACOLOGY

Amphetamines are indirect-acting sympathomimetic amines. As such they do not directly act on the receptor cells of nerve endings to bring about their effect but rather utilize the endogenous catecholamines for their actions. Many theories have been proposed for the central and peripheral effects of amphetamines, and these suggest increased liberation of endogenous catecholamine, displacement of catecholamines from binding sites, inhibition of enzymes of metabolism (monoamine oxidase), interference with reuptake, and action as a false transmitter.[1, 2, 4] The effects of amphetamines most likely are a result of a combination of these mechanisms.

Effects of the amphetamines are then understandably similar to the effects of the adrenergic transmitters and include the following:

Increased systolic and diastolic blood pressure
Increased pulse pressure
Increased heart rate (note that cardiovascular effects can be
    variable and not identical with those seen with epinephrine or norep-
    inephrine)
Relaxation of smooth muscle, e.g., bronchiolar dilatation,
    slowing of intestinal motility
Dilatation of pupils
Decreased salivary secretions
Increased metabolic rate
Increased oxygen consumption
Increased plasma-free fatty acid concentration
CNS effects, including
    increased alertness
    increase in psychomotor performance
    respiratory stimulation
    elevation of mood
    decrease in total sleep and REM sleep

These effects are variable in individuals using the drug and in the same individual with different exposures to the drug.[1,2,4,8]

Absorption of oral preparations will usually result in effects in 30 minutes. Amphetamines reach high concentration in CNS tissues, and their central effects can persist for more than 12 to 24 hours. Amphetamine metabolism follows one of several hepatic pathways: p-hydroxylation, β-hydroxylation, N-demethylation, deamination. Unchanged amphetamine as well as numerous metabolites are found in the urine.

EFFECTS ON PERFORMANCE

Numerous studies have attempted to document the effects of amphetamines on performance. [7–23] Some studies investigated psychomotor tasks,[11, 14, 21, 22] others certain variables related to performance,[7–10, 12, 13, 16, 23] and others athletic performance.[15, 17–20] In 1940 Heyrodt and Weissenstein published a study utilizing methamphetamine which showed that in runs to exhaustion, endurance could be enhanced with the use of the drugs.[13] In 1947 Cuthbertson and Knox used a single subject on a cycle ergometer to show that pedaling rate could be increased for several hours when 15 mg amphetamine sulfate was compared to a placebo.[9] The contradictory studies of Smith and Beecher[17–20] and Karpovich[15] on the effects of amphetamines on athletic performance, reported simultaneously, exemplify the confusion and contradiction found in the literature. Subsequent studies have shown positive effects on variables of performance.[8] Others have shown no effect on variables of performance.[10, 12, 13, 23] Explanations for this seeming contradiction have suggested the timing of drug administration, the dosage used, and even scientific method. Chandler and Blair concluded in 1980 that "amphetamines do not prevent fatigue but rather mask the effects of fatigue and interfere with the body's fatigue-alarm system, which could lead to disastrous results, especially under extreme environmental conditions."[8] Most will agree that the fatigued person, whether an athlete, a car or truck driver, a student, or an experimental subject, will have an increase in alertness with the use of amphetamines. They also stated that "due to the significant results for subject/treatment interaction relative to several variables, it is obvious that this drug has no consistent effects for all people, nor consistent effects when administered to the same individual on separate occasions."[8] This observation is very understandable when one considers that amphetamines are indirect-acting sympathomimetic agents whose effects are dependent on the status of the endogenous system.

ADVERSE EFFECTS

Adverse effects of drugs are normal pharmacodynamic actions that are undesirable. These can be drug-related regardless of dose, or can be dependent on dose, duration, and/or frequency. Some adverse effects of amphetamines can be seen with low doses but become more frequent at higher doses.

Central nervous system adverse effects include tremulousness, anxiety, insomnia, fever, confusion, nervousness, agitation, awareness of heart action, dry mouth, and a toxic psychosis that is marked by paranoid ideation and well-formed delusions. Deaths with the use of amphetamines have been noted owing to cerebrovascular hemorrhage, acute cardiac failure (cardiac arrhythmia), and hyperthermia. Hyperthermia is an important factor to be considered by the athlete contemplating use of amphetamines. The connection between the thermoregulatory system and amphetamines is readily understandable considering the function of catecholamines in that system.[1-4, 8, 24, 25]

As with other effects of amphetamines, the unwanted adverse effects are variable and unpredictable. In athletes who are placing a high level of stress on their physical systems, especially the cardiovascular system, the use of a substance that causes further stress can be hazardous and, in some cases, fatal.

SUMMARY

Amphetamines, which are indirect-acting sympathomimetic agents, have been used by athletes as well as other individuals in their battle with fatigue. These drugs principally affect the central nervous system, but may also affect the cardiovascular and metabolic systems (e.g., oxygen consumption, free fatty acid metabolism). Enhancement of athletic performance with amphetamines is controversial and reflects the variability seen with the use of the drug. Increases in alertness in the fatigued person are well accepted. Adverse effects include CNS effects, cardiac arrhythmias, and hyperthermia. Deaths have been reported. The use of amphetamines has been banned by the IOC. Amphetamines are detectable by currently utilized drug-testing methods.

OTHER SYMPATHOMIMETICS

Other sympathomimetic drugs that should be discussed are ephedrine and the selective β_2 agonists. Ephedrine is similar in mechanism to the amphetamines. Its clinical uses have included the nonemergency treatment of allergic reactions, asthma, hypotension during spinal anesthesia, atrioventricular block, and nasal congestion. The major use today is as a nasal decongestant. The reason for the low level of abuse centers on the intensity of anxiety and awareness of heart action experienced with its misuse or abuse.[1, 2, 26]

The β_2-agonists metaproterenol, terbutaline, and albuterol are useful in the treatment of asthma and exercise-induced bronchospasm (a condition that is estimated to affect 6 to 9 per cent of young athletes). Delivery can be via oral or inhalation routes. The advantages over less specific β-agonists are the longer duration of action, oral effectiveness, and minimal cardiac stimulation when inhaled. These medications are easily employed in a combination treatment regimen with theophylline, cromolyn, or a corticosteroid for the difficult cases.[26] The IOC allows the use of the selective β_2-agonist if notification of use is given prior to participation in competition.

CAFFEINE

HISTORY

Caffeine is a naturally occurring compound that is a plant alkaloid. It is found in the aqueous extracts *Coffea arabica* and *Cola acuminata*. The caffeine found in medications is synthetic. It is interesting that over half the world's annual production of coffee is consumed in 98 per cent of American homes, averaging 16 pounds per person.[1, 2, 27] Caffeine-containing beverages and medications are listed in Table 6–2.[1, 2, 27]

Caffeine's main clinical uses are for alertness during fatigue states, as an additive to analgesic mixtures, and as an additive in some diet pills.

PHARMACOLOGY

Caffeine is a xanthine that is a purine base. It is closely related to theobromine (a component of cocoa) and theophylline. Caffeine is rapidly absorbed after oral administration, with peak serum levels reached in 30 to 60 minutes. Caffeine has a direct effect on many areas—gastric mucosa, myocardium, medulla, reticular-activating system, blood vessels, skeletal muscle, adrenal medulla, and renal tubercles. The effects seen in these various areas include:[1, 2, 27]

1. Increased gastric acid, pepsin, and small intestine secretion.
2. Increased heart rate, stroke volume, cardiac output, and blood pressure at rest.
3. Tachyarrhythmias, both atrial and ventricular.
4. Increased lipolysis.
5. Increased contractility of skeletal muscles.
6. Increased oxygen consumption and metabolic rate.
7. Increased diuresis.

The half-life of caffeine is 3.5 hours. It is metabolized in the liver and is excreted via the kidneys unchanged or as 1-methyluric acid or 1-methylxanthine.

EFFECTS ON PERFORMANCE

Caffeine has been shown to enhance performance in endurance activities.[28–34] The proposed mechanisms for this effect include:

1. CNS stimulation
2. Increased fat metabolism
3. Increased skeletal muscle contractility.

Caffeine, like other xanthines, can increase alertness through its effects on the central nervous system. This CNS stimulation gives a decreased perception of fatigue, similar but less pronounced than that seen with the use of amphetamines.

TABLE 6–2. The Concentration of Caffeine in Common Beverages and Pharmaceuticals

Beverage or Product	Caffeine Concentration (mg/dl)	Quantity per Standard Serving Dose (mg)
Cocoa	25–30	50
Coffee	55–85	100–150
Cola drinks (other sodas also contain caffeine in smaller amounts)	10–15	35–55
Tea	55–85	100–150
Prescription Medications and Over-the-Counter Preparations	**(mg/tablet)**	
APC (aspirin/phenacetin/caffeine)	32	
Anacin	32	
Anacin—aspirin compound	32	
Cafergot	100	
Coricidin	30	
Darran compound	32	
Dristan	15	
Empirin Compound, Midol	32	
Excedrin	60–65	
Fiorinal	40	
Many cold preparations	40	
Migral	50	
No Doz	100	
Ordrinex	50	
PreMens	66	
Prolamine	140	
Spantrol	150	
Vanquish	32	
Diet Medications (Over-the Counter)	**(mg/tablet)**	Usually also contain
Anorexan	100	phenylpropanol-
Appedrine	100	amine, a sympatho-
Appress	100	mimetic agent)
Caldrin Reducing Plan	100	
Dexa Diet II	200	
Dexatrim	200	
Dietac	200	
Permathene 12	140	
Others		
Small chocolate bar	30	

From Goldfrank L, Lewin N, Melinek M, et al: Caffeine. Hosp Phys 43:42–59, 1981.

The substrates that are utilized as fuel for endurance activities are mainly free fatty acids and muscle glycogen. The longer the muscle glycogen is "spared," the greater the delay in the onset of exhaustion.[32] Through the increased plasma levels of free fatty acids with caffeine ingestion, these substances will be utilized as fuel, and the muscle glycogen stores will not be depleted as rapidly. Caffeine seems to affect glycogenolysis and inhibit utilization of muscle glycogen stores.[30–33]

Caffeine has been shown to have a direct effect on the skeletal muscle contractile properties. Significant increases in muscle tension in the adductor pollucis muscle were found by Lopes et al. when caffeine was ingested in both nonfatigued and fatigued states.[35] This may also contribute to the enhancement of performance seen with caffeine. This enhancement is limited to endurance activities, however. Maximal exercise bouts for short periods are not significantly improved by caffeine.[36]

Caffeine is banned by the IOC in amounts greater than 15µg/ml in the urine.

ADVERSE EFFECTS

Caffeine is also associated with unwanted adverse effects. Many of these are dose-related, with symptoms such as headache, tremors, nervousness, diuresis, and arrhythmias (tachycardias) possibly occurring in the 200- to 500-mg range and increasing in incidence as the dose is increased to the 750-mg range.

The most common adverse effects are CNS related and include restlessness, tremulousness, hyperactivity, irritability, dry mouth, dysesthesias, tinnitus, ocular dyskinesia, scotomata, myalgias, insomnia, headaches, and depression. Goldfrank et al.[27] present the five-symptom cluster of CNS involvement from caffeinism. These include:

1. Anxiety-like presentation
2. Hypochondriasis-like presentation
3. Insomnia and/or headache presentation
4. Withdrawal symptoms
5. Depressive presentation

The effects of caffeine on the myocardium include increases in the sinus rate, ectopic beats, and force of contraction. Caffeine can be a factor in those who experience paroxysmal atrial tachycardia (PAT), and removal of caffeine may be the sole necessary therapy in some individuals. Caffeine has also been associated with exacerbation of migraine headaches.[1, 2, 27, 37]

There is a withdrawal syndrome described for those who are regular users of significant amounts of caffeine daily. The syndrome includes headache, drowsiness, lethargy, rhinorrhea, irritability, nervousness, depressive feelings, and disinclination to work.[27]

Caffeine also has a diuretic effect, which may produce problems for those involved in activities where maintenance of hydration is important and difficult.

SUMMARY

Caffeine, a xanthine, is used by athletes principally in endurance events. The ability of caffeine to increase free fatty acid utilization, to mask fatigue through CNS stimulation, and to increase the force of contraction of skeletal muscle makes it an attractive drug to the endurance athlete. The adverse effects are seen primarily on the central nervous and cardiovascular systems and include hyperactivity, irritability, restlessness, insomnia, and arrhythmias. Caffeine is banned by the IOC if urine values are greater than 15 μg/ml.

COCAINE

HISTORY

Cocaine is not a new drug but an old drug that has found new popularity. It occurs naturally in the leaf of the *Erythroxylon coca* plant. The coca leaf had a sacred status in the time of the Incas and was utilized in rituals by the priests of the tribe. In the sixth century, it was reportedly used by Peruvian natives to aid their work at high altitudes. In the nineteenth century, Gaedcke isolated the first coca extract and Niemann isolated the principal active ingredient. Sigmund Freud used cocaine therapeutically as a stimulant, for digestive disorders, for other drug addictions, for asthma, and as a local anesthetic.[38–40] The property of local anesthesia, the only true therapeutic value of the drug, was utilized by Koller, Halsted, Jelliner, and Corning.

Vin Mariani, a coca-containing elixir, was produced by the Corsican chemist Angelo Mariani and was a "cure-all" that was used by many famous and respected individuals including Thomas Edison, William McKinley, Pope Leo XIII, Jules Verne, Auguste Rodin, H.G. Wells, and Henrik Ibsen. Coca-Cola had cocaine in its original formula, but this was removed from the soft drink in 1903. Between 1900 and 1920, cocaine fell into disfavor because of its potential for developing dependency in users and its association with crime. Cocaine has again become popular as a recreational drug. The business of cocaine growing, processing, transporting, selling, and buying produces billions of dollars of revenue each year.[37–39]

The history of cocaine is especially interesting for two reasons. It shows, first, that people do not learn from the lessons of the past and, second, that the controlling effects of the drug are not limited by intellect, success, talent, or money.

PHARMACOLOGY

Cocaine is a natural alkaloid that can be extracted from the coca leaf and purified to the hydrochloride salt. The main actions of cocaine are:

1. Local anesthesia
2. Stimulation of central nervous system
3. Cardiorespiratory stimulation

The methods of cocaine entry used by abusers include:

1. Sniffing—inhaling the crystals through a straw or rolled-up bill. it is absorbed via the nasal mucosa, and the "high" is rapid in onset, peaking in about 20 minutes.

2. Smoking
   a. Coca paste (a less pure form of cocaine) smoking—The onset of action is rapid, and duration of "high" is short.
   b. Freebase smoking—smoking of the extract of basic cocaine prepared with the use of a volatile solvent such as ether. Many accidental burns have been reported. Very rapid onset with intense "rush" and euphoria lasting only a few minutes.
3. Intravenous—a very dangerous method of taking the drug owing to the rapid onset of effect, varying concentrations of cocaine, and different adulterants with which cocaine is cut (Peak: 3 to 5 minutes).

Metabolism of cocaine occurs quickly, with a majority (80 per cent) excreted in the urine within 24 hours. The two main urinary metabolites of cocaine are benzoylecgonine and ecgonine methylester.[38–40]

Cocaine is a potent reinforcer of behavior in animal research. If permitted, monkeys will continually self-inject and increase doses of cocaine in lieu of eating, drinking, sleeping, and sex.[38] This correlates well with the statements of cocaine abusers that cocaine becomes the most important aspect of their life.

EXTENT OF PROBLEM

Many estimates have been made as to the extent of the cocaine explosion in society. Estimates have been made that 28 per cent of adults between 20 and 40 years of age have tried cocaine. It is estimated that 16 per cent of high school seniors have tried cocaine and that 0.2 per cent use the drug regularly. Athletes, because of their public presence and financial status in society, are targets of cocaine distributors. Cocaine use has been glamorized by the public.[41]

Reports of cocaine problems among athletes are regularly in the newspapers. The effect of such drug use is detrimental not only to the individual athlete but also to the younger athletes for whom he or she serves as a role model or idol. The habits of "famous" individuals have a tendency to trickle down through colleges, high schools, and elementary schools. It is felt that as availability increases and/or price decreases, the problem of cocaine abuse will grow at all levels.

ADVERSE EFFECTS

The adverse effects of cocaine center on the central nervous system and the cardiorespiratory system. Effects that may impair athletic performance include:

1. Accelerated mental processes
2. Euphoria
3. Feelings of increased mental and physical power
4. Paranoia

Cocaine overdose can lead to arrhythmias, coma, seizures, hyperthermia, and death.[42–44] The treatment of these problems is difficult when they occur in an adequately staffed medical facility. When overdose occurs in the street or at a party, the prognosis is poor. The best method of caring for the acute overdose in the field is to administer cardiopulmonary resuscitation if necessary and immediately take the victim to a hospital. The use of cocaine can result in tremulousness, agitation, restlessness, insomnia, and anxiety, as with any other stimulant. A toxic psychosis is associated with cocaine and is characterized by hallucinations (auditory, visual, or olfactory), paranoia (especially of the police), and delusions (itching from "parasites" under the skin).[45] Frequent nosebleeds or chronic rhinitis can be seen with septal necrosis in some chronic cocaine users. Cocaine also can alter the thermoregulatory system, which can be extremely hazardous for the athlete exercising in hot and humid climates. A withdrawal syndrome characterized by irritability, depression, suicidal ideation, and a strong desire for the drug can be seen.[45]

Some behavioral changes one might see in a user of cocaine include:

1. Late for or missed appointments
2. Loner tendency, especially on trips
3. Missed assignments
4. Lack of attention at meetings
5. Financial difficulties
6. Personal problems

These should identify that the athlete is having a problem that is placing him or her under a great deal of stress. Remember that the problem may be chemical(drug)-related.

TREATMENT

Many treatment plans have been instituted for chemical dependency. The treatment is best delivered by those who regularly deal with this problem. The treatment plan includes:

1. Identification of the problem through signs and symptoms, legal entanglement, drug screening; and acceptance of the problem.
2. Withdrawal of the drug as an inpatient or outpatient, as deemed necessary by a specialist.
3. Therapy—Individual, group, and support group (e.g., Cocaine Anonymous) therapies are keys to the successful avoidance of recurrent cocaine use. Testing for "cleanliness" (drug freedom) is accomplished with regular observed urine checks. The clearance of cocaine from the urine is about three days, so urine checks must be scheduled accordingly.

A model of drug treatment in the professional athlete is the "Inner Circle" of the Cleveland Browns professional football team. This concept of a team's approach to the problem of chemical dependency requires a tremendous commitment of time, energy, and finances of all involved. It has been successful in dealing with the problem.

Many treatment centers realize both short- and long-term success.

For the best hope of recovery, it is important to enlist the aid of an individual who regularly treats chemical dependency.

SUMMARY

Cocaine, a naturally occurring alkaloid, has a long history of use for medicinal, religious, and recreational reasons. The local anesthetic, central stimulatory and cardiorespiratory stimulatory effects produce the user's desired "high" as well as the physical and psychological adverse effects. Treatment should be conducted by those familiar with chemical dependency, but identification of the problem is the responsibility of all.

NICOTINE

HISTORY

Nicotine has been utilized by many cultures in various ways. In European culture, smoking became prevalent after the discovery of the New World. In Australia, the aborigines chewed leaves containing a nicotine-like substance. American Indians smoked a leaf containing lobeline, which has properties similar to nicotine. Chewing tobacco or smoking rolled tobacco became popular in the "Old West."[1, 2]

National Institute of Drug Abuse surveys report that in 1982, 70 per cent of high school seniors had tried smoking cigarettes and 21.1 per cent were daily users. These figures have decreased since the peak year of 1977 when 76 per cent tried and 28.8 per cent were daily users.[41] Remington reports decreasing trends among all groups in cigarette smoking. However, between 1965 and 1982 there was a 17 per cent decrease (51 to 34 per cent) in adult male smokers, while only a 4 per cent decrease (33 to 29 per cent) in adult female smokers.[46] The education process concerning smoking and emphasizing the risks has seemingly affected the advertising campaigns of the tobacco companies.

An increase has been seen in the use of "smokeless" tobacco, which is also known as "chew." It has been reported that in Texas up to one third of varsity football and baseball players are using smokeless tobacco. Advertisers have projected that in the next decade there will be a doubling of the estimated 22 million current users.[47]

The use of nicotine, both smoked and chewed, remains high among all groups of society, whether athletes or nonathletes. In other areas, nicotine is used as an insecticide and in laboratory investigations as an inducer of convulsions.

PHARMACOLOGY

Nicotine is an alkaloid that exerts effects on both the sympathetic and parasympathetic nervous systems. Nicotine uses the same mechanism as acetylcholines to effect sympathetic stimulation—stimulation of adrenal medulla; facilitation of transmission across sympathetic ganglia; and causing norepinephrine release from cardiac atria and arterioles. Due to the effects on various cardiovascular control centers (e.g., carotid and aortic bodies), the sympathetic and vagal ganglia, and the cardiac muscle, bradycardia or occasionally tachycardia and elevation of blood pressure can be seen with nicotine use. Parasympathomimetic stimulation also occurs via muscarinic receptors causing increases in gastrointestinal muscle tone and peristaltic movement. Pupillary constriction can also be seen. Antidiuretic hormone is released from the posterior lobe of the pituitary, resulting in decreased urine volume. Nicotine also increases the secretion of saliva, bronchial mucus, and sweat. The satiety center of the brain is stimulated by nicotine, which may explain the weight gain associated with smoking cessation.[1, 2]

Nicotine is well absorbed through the lungs, mucous membranes, and all body surfaces. The rate of absorption is faster through the lungs than through the mucous membranes.

EFFECTS ON PERFORMANCE

Some athletes use nicotine for the stimulating effect prior to their event. Others reportedly use the tobacco for the seemingly paradoxical calming effect prior to competition. Also there are those who use nicotine for its effect on the satiety center for weight control. Finally, there are those athletes who have no performance-related reason for tobacco use.

Some studies have shown the effect of smoking on various parameters related to performance. Rode and Shephard reported the oxygen cost of ventilation (energy necessary to breathe) was higher in smokers than nonsmokers during vigorous exercise.[48, 49] Sepponen showed a decrease in physical work capacity and an increase in heart rate after cigarette smoking.[50] Klausen et al. found that acutely, smoking results in increased resting heart rate, decreased maximal heart rate, and decreased maximum oxygen uptake during maximal exercise testing.[51] Maksud and Baron found that smokers had more increased minute ventilations during submaximal exercise and higher perceived exertion than nonsmokers. However, they found no difference in aerobic power (maximum oxygen uptake) or physical work capacity in their study of blue collar workers.[52]

Butts and Golding concluded that after 24 hours of smoking cessation, improvements can be seen in cardiac efficiency in chronic smokers.[53] This suggests that some improvement in physiological parameters can be seen in even chronic smokers if they abstain for one full day.

Markiewicz et al. found better utilization of free fatty acids during physical exertion after previous tobacco smoking owing to the effects of nicotine.[54]

Timisjarvi, by using radiocardiography to study the effects of smoking on the central circulation, concluded that smoking impairs physical performance. Significant increases in heart rate and pulmonary capillary pressure were found with a reduction in pulmonary blood volume.[55]

Bal and White surveyed college students concerning general health and sleeping patterns and found that smokers had a higher incidence of minor health problems and slept less and poorly when compared with nonsmokers.[56] This could hamper performance, since fatigue, the athlete's worst enemy, is difficult to defeat without proper sleep.

The studies show effects on various physiological parameters that contribute to athletic performance. Some may be viewed as positive or at least not negative, but most effects of smoking/nicotine must be viewed as detrimental to the performance of the athlete.

Unfortunately, there is a paucity of studies performed on the effects of chewing tobacco on parameters affecting performance. Considering the great increase in smokeless tobacco, this would be an interesting and important avenue of research.

Adverse Effects

As detrimental as smoking potentially is to athletic performance, its association with serious disease is more significant. In 1982, the surgeon general reported that "cigarette smoking is the chief preventable cause of death in our society."[57]

In 1950, Wynder and Graham suggested the connection between tobacco smoking and bronchogenic carcinoma.[58] This has been supported by many since that early article. The American Cancer Society projects that more American women will die of lung cancer than breast cancer by the end of the 1980's. Lung cancer remains the leading cause of cancer-associated deaths (87,000) among American men.[59] Smoking has been associated with increased prevalence of coronary artery disease, subsequent myocardial infarction, and sudden death.[60, 61] It is considered a major risk factor in the development of coronary artery disease. There has been an association between cigarette smoking and the development of chronic obstructive pulmonary disease[60, 61] as well as acute respiratory tract illness.[62] Cigarette smoking was shown to be associated with delayed conception by smoking women.[63]

Chewing tobacco is associated with oral, pharyngeal, and laryngeal cancers. It also is associated with dental problems (receding gums, tooth decay, etc.), leukoplakia (plaque development on the oral mucosa which can be a precursor of cancer), and decreased taste and smell sensitivity.

The adverse effects of the nicotine contained in tobacco that is smoked or chewed are many and serious. Nicotine itself is associated with cardiac arrhythmias, convulsions, and death when taken in toxic doses.[1, 2] The strong desire for or dependence on smoking is felt to be due to a dependence on nicotine. This is demonstrated by the difficulty encountered by those who attempt to stop smoking and the poor results of many "stop smoking" efforts.[57]

Summary

Nicotine is used by a significant number of individuals. This stimulant is taken in the smoked form of a cigarette or the chewed form of smokeless tobacco. Smoking has been shown to negatively affect physiological parameters of exercise performance. Smokeless tobacco needs further study in the area of effect on performance. The risks of both smoking and chewing are significant in the development of cardiovascular, pulmonary, and oral diseases. Smoking and chewing are difficult habits to break, and prevention by abstinence is the best approach.

REFERENCES

1. Crossland J: Lewis' Pharmacology, 5th ed. New York, Churchill Livingstone, 1980, pp. 83–96, 258–286.
2. Meyers FH, Jawetz E, Goldfein A: Review of Medical Pharmacology, 6th ed. Los Altos, CA, Lange Medical Publications, 1979, pp 79–93, 294–306.
3. Smith DE (ed): Amphetamine Use, Misuse and Abuse: Proceedings of the National Amphetamine Conference, 1978. Boston, G.K. Hall and Company, 1979, pp 18–21.
4. Morgan JF: Clinical Pharmacology of Amphetamines. In Smith DE (ed): Amphetamine Use, Misuse and Abuse: Proceedings of the National Amphetamine Conference, 1978. Boston, G.K. Hall and Company, 1979, pp 3–10.
5. Mandell AJ: The Sunday syndrome: A unique pattern of amphetamine abuse indigenous to American professional football. Clin Toxicol 15(2):225–232, 1979.
6. Blyth CS, Allen M, Lovingood BW: Effects of amphetamine (Dexedrine) and caffeine on subjects exposed to heat and exercise stress. Res Q 31(4):553–559, 1960.
7. Laties VG, Weiss B: The amphetamine margin in sports. Fed Proc 40 (12):2689–2692, October 1981.
8. Chandler JB, Blair VS: The effect of amphetamines on selected physiological components related to athletic success. Med Sci Sports Exer 12(1):65–69, 1980.
9. Cuthbertson DP, Knox JAC: The effects of analeptics on the fatigued subject. J Physiol (Lond) 106:42–58, 1947.
10. Golding LA, Barnard JR: The effect of delta amphetamine sulfate on physical performance. J Sports Med 19:221–224, 1963.
11. Goldstein A, Searle BW, Schimke RT: Effects of secobarbital and of delta amphetamine on psychomotor performance of normal subjects. J Pharmacol Exp Ther 130: 55–58, 1960.
12. Haldi J, Wynn W: Action of drugs on efficiency of swimmers. Res Q 17:96–101, 1946.
13. Heyrodt H, Weissenstein J: Uber Steigerung Korperlicher Leistungfahigkeit durch Pervitin. Arch Exp Pathol Pharmakol 195:273–275, 1940.
14. Holliday AR, Divery WJ: Effects of drugs on the performance of a task by fatigued subjects. Clin Pharmacol Ther 3:(1) 5–15, 1963.
15. Karpovich PV: Effect of amphetamine sulfate on athletic performance. JAMA 170(5):558–561, 1969.
16. Lovingood BW, Blyth CS, Peacock WH, et al: Effects of delta-amphetamine sulfate, caffeine and high temperature on human performance. Res Q 38:(1):64–71, 1967.
17. Smith GM, Beecher HK: Amphetamine sulfate and athletic performance. JAMA 170(5):542–557, 1959.
18. Smith GM, Beecher HK: Amphetamine, secobarbital and athletic performance. JAMA 172(14): 1502–1514, 1960.
19. Smith GM, Beecher HK: Amphetamine, secobarbital and athletic performance. JAMA 172(15):1623–1629, 1960.
20. Smith GM, Weitzner M, Beecher HK: Increased sensitivity of measurement of drug effects in expert swimmers. J Pharmacol Exp Ther 139:114–119, 1963.
21. Thornton GR, Holck HG, Smith EL: The effect of Benzedrine and caffeine upon performance in certain psychomotor tasks. J Abnorm Soc Psychol 96–113, 1939.
22. Tyler DB: The effect of amphetamine sulfate and some barbiturates on the fatigue produced by prolonged wakefulness. Am J Physiol 150:253–262, 1947.
23. Williams MH, Thompson J: Effect of variant dosages of amphetamine upon endurance. Res Q 44 (4):417–422, 1973.
24. Kalant H, Kalant, OJ: Death in amphetamine users: Cause and rates. In Smith DE (ed):

Amphetamine Use, Misuse and Abuse: Proceedings of the National Amphetamine Conference, 1978. Boston, G.K. Hall and Company, 1979, pp 169–188.

25. Snyder S: Amphetamine psychosis: A "model schizophrenia" medicated by catecholamines. In Smith DE (ed): Amphetamine Use, Misuse and Abuse: Proceedings of the National Amphetamine Conference, 1978. Boston, G.K. Hall and Company, 1979, pp 189–204.

26. Sly RM: Beta-adrenergic drugs in management of asthma in athletes. J Allergy Clin Immunol 73:680–685, May 1984.

27. Goldfrank L, Lewin N, Melinek M, et al: Caffeine. Hosp Phys 43:42–59, 1981.

28. Barta L, Pena M, Tichy M, et al: The effect of caffeine and physical exercise on blood lactate levels of obese children. Acta Paediatr Acad Sci Hung 23:343–347, 1982.

29. Berglund B, Hemmingsson P: Effects of caffeine ingestion on exercise performance at low and high altitudes in cross country skiers. Int J Sports Med 2:234–236, 1982.

30. Essig D, Costill DL, Van Handel PJ: Effects of caffeine ingestion on utilization of muscle glycogen and lipid during leg ergometer cycling. Int J Sports Med 1:86–90, 1980.

31. Costill DL, Dalsky GP, Fink WJ: Effects of caffeine ingestion on metabolism and exercise performance. Med Sci Sports 19(3):155–158, 1978.

32. Ivy JL, Costill DL, Fink WJ, et al: Influence of caffeine and carbohydrate feedings on endurance performance. Med Sci Sports 11(1):6–11, 1979.

33. Toner MM, Kirkendall DT, Delio DJ, et al: Metabolic and cardiovascular responses to exercise with caffeine. Ergonomics 25(2):1175–1183, 1982.

34. Wilcox AR: The effects of caffeine and exercise on body weight, fat pad weight and fat cell size. Med Sci Sports Exerc 14(4):317–321, 1982.

35. Lopes JM, Jardin J, Aubier M, Aranda JV, Macklem PT: Effect of caffeine on skeletal muscle function before and after fatigue. J Appl Physiol 54(5):1303–1305, May 1983.

36. Van Handel PJ: Effects of caffeine on physical performance. J Phys Ed Rec, February 1980, pp 56–57.

37. Onrot J, Biaggion I, Hollister A, et al: The cardiovascular effects of caffeine. Primary Cardiol, October 1984, pp 104–110.

38. Smith DE: The Coke Book. New York, Berkley Books, 1984.

39. Petersen RC, Cohen S, Jeri FR, et al: Cocaine: A second look. American Council on Marijuana and Other Psychoactive Drugs, Inc., 1983.

40. Gold MS: 800-Cocaine. Toronto, Bantam Books, June 1984.

41. National Institute on Drug Abuse. National Survey on Drug Abuse: Main Findings, 1982. U.S. Department of Health and Human Services. Public Health Service. Alcohol, Drug Abuse and Mental Health Administration. Rockville, MD, DHHS Publication No. (ADM), 1983, pp 83–1263.

42. Wetli CV, Wright RK: Death caused by recreational cocaine use. JAMA 241 (23):2519–2522, June 1979.

43. Alfred RJ, Ewer S: Case report: Fatal pulmonary edema following intravenous "freebase" cocaine use. Ann Emerg Med 10(8):441, August 1981.

44. Fishbain DA, Wetli CV: Case report: Cocaine intoxication, delirium, and death in a body packer. Ann Emerg Med 10(10):531–532, October 1981.

45. Collins GB: Clues to cocaine dependency. Diagnosis, January 1985, pp 57–65.

46. Remington PL, Forman MR, Gentry EM, et al: Current smoking trends in the United States. The 1981–1983 behavioral risk factor surveys. JAMA 253(20):2975–2978, 1985.

47. Moran M: Smokeless tobacco is "burning" young athletes. Phys Sports Med 9(3):21, 1981.

48. Rode A, Shephard R: The influence of cigarette smoking upon the oxygen cost of breathing in near maximal exercise. Med Sci Sports 3(2):51–55, 1971.

49. Shephard R: The oxygen cost of breathing during vigorous exercise. Q J Exp Physiol 51:336–350, 1966.

50. Sepponen A: Physical work capacity in relation to carbon monoxide inhalation and tobacco smoking. Ann Clin Res 9:269–274, 1977.

51. Klausen K, Andersen S, Nandrup S: Acute effects of cigarette smoking and inhalation of carbon monoxide during maximal exercise. Eur J Appl Physiol 51:371–379, 1983.

52. Maksud MC, Baron A: Physiological responses to exercise in chronic cigarette and marijuana users. Eur J Appl Physiol 43:127–134, 1980.
53. Butts, NK, Golding LA: Effects of 24 hours of smoking withdrawal on cardiorespiratory function at rest and exercise. J Sports Med 19:389–396, 1979.
54. Markiewicz K, Cholewa M, Luciak M: Influence of tobacco smoking on serum free fatty acids, triglycerides and glucose levels during physical training and post-exertional restitution. Acta Med Acad Sci Hung Tom 35:3–4, 225–232, 1978.
55. Timisjarvi J, Kuikka L, Hirvonen R, et al: Effect of smoking on the central circulation at rest and during exercise as studied by radiocardiography. Nuclear Med 19(5)239–243, 1980.
56. Ball P, White M: The effects of smoking on the health and sleep of sportswomen. Br J Sports Med 16(3):149–153, 1982.
57. New knowledge about nicotine effects. Medical News (editorial). JAMA 247(17):2333–2338, 1982.
58. Wynder EL, Graham EA: Tobacco smoking as a possible etiologic factor in bronchogenic carcinoma. JAMA 143:329–336, 1950.
59. Seeking to end smoking's appeal to women, youth. Medical News (editorial). JAMA 253(20):2943–2944, 1985.
60. Smoking and Health. Report of the Advisory Committee to the Surgeon General of the Public Health Service. Publication 1103, Public Health Service, 1974.
61. Smoking and Health. Report of the Surgeon General. U.S. Department of Health, Education and Welfare. Public Health Service, January 11, 1979.
62. Aronson M, Weiss ST, Beh, RL et al: Association between cigarette smoking and acute respiratory tract illness in young adults. JAMA 248(2):181–183, 1982.
63. Baird DD, Wilcox AJ: Cigarette smoking associated with delayed conception. JAMA 253(20):2979–2983, 1985.

7

DEPRESSANTS

JOHN A. LOMBARDO, M.D.

High self-expectations, peer and team expectations, family's and friends' expectations, and fans' expectations can contribute to increased anxiety levels before, during, and after performance. Some athletes find relief in activities outside their event; some turn to psychotherapy or relaxation therapy; others find escape from their fears in chemicals.

The depressants, or downers, are predominantly used as relaxants. Alcohol, marijuana, sedatives, barbiturates, and beta blockers are used to calm. In some instances the drugs are taken prior to an event, but most frequently these are used as relaxants after the game or match.

ALCOHOL

HISTORY

Ethyl alcohol has been used as a beverage, potion, anesthetic, or means of escape in different cultures through the ages. Fermentation of fruit juices, sap, or grain produces alcohol concentrations in the ranges of 14 to 16 per cent. Through the process of distilling, more concentrated or stronger liquors can be produced.[1] The concentrations of alcohol in different beverages are beer 2 to 6 per cent, wines 12 to 20 per cent, and distilled liquors 35 to 50 per cent.[1]

The National Institute of Drugs and Alcohol (NIDA) surveyed high school seniors and reported that in 1982, 93 per cent of seniors had tried alcohol, 70 per cent had used alcohol in the month prior to the survey, and 5.7 per cent were daily users of alcohol. In the 18 to 25 age range, 7 per cent used alcohol daily in 1982. The age group of 26 and over reported 11.4 per cent daily users.[2]

Alcohol abuse is a problem in every age group. Athletes were once felt to be immune to the evils of alcohol and drug use. However, recent revelations have shown that modern athletes in high school, college, and professional ranks are exposed to the same risks as the general population. Published reports describing the antics of athletes of past eras indicate that alcohol played a large part in the lives of some of these legends of sport.

Therapeutically, alcohol has been used as an anesthetic for surgical procedures when no other agent was available (as in old western films). It is also an excellent solvent and is used in the preparation of tinctures, solutions (such as cough syrups), and extracts. Alcohol has been given intravenously to slow premature labor contractions. In individuals with painful neuralgias, alcohol has been injected in the area of the involved nerve. Most of these uses for alcohol have been discontinued with the development of other methods and substances.[1, 3]

PHARMACOLOGY

Alcohol is absorbed in the stomach (up to 20 per cent) and the small intestines (remainder). Ninety per cent of a single dose is absorbed in an hour, and peak blood level is reached in 40 to 45 minutes.[3] Alcohol is then distributed throughout the body in proportion to the water content of the tissue. In the liver, alcohol is oxidized to acetaldehyde, which is then further oxidized in the liver and other tissues containing aldehyde dehydrogenase.[1] Disulfiram (Antabuse) interferes with the oxidation of acetaldehyde, thereby raising levels of acetaldehyde in individuals who drink alcohol while taking the drug. This produces acetaldehyde toxicity, which results in flushing, vertigo, hypotension, headache, excessive sweating, nausea, vomiting, and abdominal pain.[4]

If allowed to continue uninterrupted, the oxidation of alcohol is a zero-order reaction (a constant amount metabolized regardless of amount present), and 10 to 15 ml per hour is metabolized.[3]

Alcohol diffusely depresses the central nervous sytem, which results in a number of changes that are related to the amount of alcohol in the system.

Table 7–1 gives an example of the effects of varying amounts of alcohol on blood alcohol levels and behavior.

EFFECTS ON PERFORMANCE

Many stories have been told concerning the accomplishments of an individual either while intoxicated or the day after an alcoholic binge. There are also many athletes who have had major accomplishments despite being chronic alcohol abusers. These isolated instances do not make a case for the general use of alcohol as an enhancer of performance.

Many studies have been performed concerning the various aspects of performance and the use of alcohol. The benefits of improving self-

TABLE 7–1. Effects of Alcohol Consumption on Blood Levels and Behavior

Blood Alcohol Concentration (mg/dl)	Amount of Alcohol Needed		State
	DOUBLE WHISKEY	PINTS OF BEER	
50	1	1	Euphoria, minor motor disturbances
60			Nystagmus, more errors on simple tests
80	1½	2	Impaired driving ability, EEG changes
100–150	2–3	3–4	Gross motor incoordination
200–300	4–6	6–9	Mobile, but amnesia for the experience
300–350	6–7	9–10	Coma
350–600	7–12	11–18	Coma, may cause death

Adapted from Meyers FH, Jawetz E, Goldfien A (eds): Review of Medical Pharmacology, 6th ed. Los Altos, CA, Lange Medical Publications, 1978, and Crossland J: Lewis' Pharmacology, 5th ed. New York, Churchill Livingstone, 1980.

confidence and relaxation[5] are far outweighed by the adverse effects or impairment of the following functions:

1. Reaction time [6-10] (essential for optimal performance).
2. Hand-eye coordination[10-12] (decreased capacity in this area can result in not only less than optimum performance but also injury, especially in sports in which a projectile is used).
3. Accuracy[8, 13] (another factor that is important in target-related events such as archery and riflery and in goal-directed sports such as soccer and baseball).
4. Balance[14] (a much underrated and often forgotten factor in many sports—important in apparatus events such as gymnastics and also in jumping sports such as volleyball and basketball).
5. Complex coordination of gross motor skills[8, 10, 15, 16] (this is the area in which many great athletes are set apart from the less accomplished).

Psychomotor functions undergo significant changes with alcohol use. These functions, as noted above, are of paramount importance to any athlete trying to perform his or her best at a particular activity.

Two of the parameters of conditioning—strength and endurance—have been studied. In the area of muscular strength, some studies have shown no effect of alcohol,[17-20] while others have shown that a decrease in strength may result from the use of alcohol.[8, 19, 21] There is therefore no benefit to be gained in the area of muscular strength by the use of alcohol. The only significant changes shown were decreases—a negative factor for the athlete.

Endurance, or aerobic capacity, is another parameter that has been studied for the effects of alcohol. Oxygen uptake has been shown to be unaffected by alcohol in all but one study using submaximal work and in all the studies using maximal work.[22-26] Thus, the literature supports the contention that alcohol has no effect on the aerobic capacity of man.

Alcohol's overall effect on performance of exercise and sports is detrimental. When the negative effects on psychomotor function, potential negative effects on muscular strength, and lack of effect on aerobic capacity are weighed against the potential gain in self-confidence and relaxation, the scales tip to the negative side.

ADVERSE EFFECTS

Alcohol is associated with many adverse effects. The legality of the use of alcohol is mistakenly thought by some to represent the safety of alcohol.

Alcohol is the number one drug of abuse in the United States. The survey by NIDA showed that 6.5 per cent of young adults (18 to 25 years old) and 11.4 per cent of older adults (age 26 and above) used alcohol for 20 or more days in the month prior to the survey. Also, interestingly, 28.2 per cent of the young adults and 18.2 per cent of the older adults used alcohol 5 to 19 days of the month prior to the survey. Alcohol drinkers also have a higher incidence of use of other drugs—e.g., marijuana, cocaine, etc.—than nondrinkers.[2] Alcoholism claims approximately 13 million Americans, over 3 million of whom are in the 14 to 17 age group.[27] It is certainly a problem with which the population must deal.

Alcoholic cardiomyopathy is a dilated cardiomyopathy. Alcoholics have been shown to have elevated left ventricular wall stress and an exaggerated stress-to-mass ratio. Abnormalities of systolic time intervals and lower left ventricular ejection phase indices were also found in a group of alcoholics when compared to a matched normal population.[28]

Even though early studies showed a seemingly dose-related protective effect of alcohol against coronary artery disease by lowering serum HDL-C, these studies lacked the ability to fractionate HDL-C.[28] Subsequent studies have shown HDL-C levels to be higher with up to two ounces of alcohol per day, but the fraction that is elevated is not the fraction associated with coronary artery disease reduction.[29] Individuals who imbibe larger quantities regularly—the problem drinker—have been found to have a high risk of developing coronary artery disease and also an increased risk of cerebrovascular accidents.[28]

Blood pressure is another area affected by alcohol intake. Elevated blood pressure is noted with larger amounts of alcohol, whereas moderate use of alcohol may lower blood pressure.[28]

Alcohol has been shown to affect the fetus during pregnancy. Maternal alcohol consumption has been shown to correlate with low-birth weight, lower weight being associated with increasing amounts of alcohol.[30] This is one of the elements of the fetal alcohol syndrome found in the offspring of alcoholic mothers.[31, 32]

Alcohol can affect sexual function in a negative manner in both men and women. Impotence and organic dysfunction as well as the crimes of rape and pedophilia have been associated with alcohol use.[33, 34]

Neurologically, the chronic alcohol user has demonstrated peripheral neuropathy, Wernicke's disease (impaired eye movements, ataxic gait, mental confusion), Korsakoff's psychosis (amnestic confabulation), and cerebellar degeneration (ataxic gait and leg and trunk ataxia). All of these problems are related to vitamin deficiencies, predominantly thiamine deficiency.[35]

Half of all traffic fatalities and one third of all traffic injuries are alcohol-related.[36] Twenty-four of 30 drivers killed in snowmobile accidents were driving under the influence of alcohol.[37] Alcohol has been shown to be a factor in death by drowning in a number of studies.[38–40]

The damage to the gastrointestinal tract ranges from irritation of the gastric mucosa from gastritis to ulceration, alcohol-induced pancreatitis, and liver damage from fatty infiltration to cirrhosis.[41, 42]

Heavy use of alcohol has been identified as a factor in the development of oropharyngeal, laryngeal, esophageal, and primary hepatocellular carcinoma.[43]

Alcohol has also been shown to produce hypoglycemia and increased heat loss when an individual exercises mildly in a cold environment.[44] This can result in difficulty regulating body temperature. This is an interesting effect, since some believe alcohol is an antifreeze that helps cope with the cold.

Identification of the Problem Drinker

One of the difficult problems in dealing with the alcohol-abusing patient is identifying the problem. The symptoms of an adolescent with a chemical dependency (alcohol- or drug-related) include:

1. Sudden, noticeable personality changes
2. Severe mood swings
3. Changing peer groups
4. Dropping out of extracurricular activities
5. Decreased interest in leisure-time activity
6. Worsening grades
7. Irresponsible attitudes toward household jobs and curfews
8. Depressed feelings much of the time
9. Dramatic change in personal hygiene
10. Changes in sleeping or eating habits
11. Smell of alcohol or marijuana
12. Sudden weight loss
13. Tendency toward increasing dishonesty
14. Trouble with the law: driving while intoxicated, possession of illegal drugs, theft, etc.
15. Truancy from school
16. Frequent job losses or changes
17. "Turned off" attitude if drugs are discussed

18. Missing household money or objects
19. Increasing time alone in his or her room
20. Deteriorating family relationships
21. Drug use paraphernalia, booze, or empty bottles found hidden
22. Observations by other people of negative behavior in the adolescent
23. Obvious signs of physical intoxication

These symptoms can also be seen in adult alcohol abusers.

Another helpful tool is the CAGE Questionnaire, which includes the following questions:

1. Have you ever felt you ought to **C**ut down on your drinking?
2. Have people **A**nnoyed you by criticizing your drinking?
3. Have you ever felt bad or **G**uilty about your drinking?
4. Have you ever had a drink first thing in the morning to steady your nerves or get rid of a hangover (**E**ye-opener)?[45]

Positive responses are not diagnostic of alcohol abuse but should raise a yellow flag and add alcohol use to the differential diagnosis.

SUMMARY

Alcohol is the most abused drug in the United States. The use of alcohol crosses all aspects of our society. On the positive side, the effects of alcohol on performance include relaxation and relief of anxiety. On the negative side is the impairment of reaction time, hand-eye coordination, accuracy, balance, and complex coordination of gross motor skills. Adverse effects include cardiovascular changes, fetal changes with maternal use, sexual dysfunction, neurological changes, increased incidence of accidents, gastrointestinal changes, association with cancer, and changes in the thermoregulatory system.

A knowledge of the warning signs as well as an awareness of the possibility of alcohol abuse as a problem are necessary to identify the problem drinker.

MARIJUANA

HISTORY

Marijuana is an ancient medicinal herb first reported in 2737 B.C. by Shen Nung, a Chinese emperor. It was used as an analgesic, anticonvulsant, sedative-hypnotic, topical anesthetic, muscle relaxant, appetite-stimulant, and bronchodilator through the centuries in Asia, Africa, and South America. Marijuana was introduced to Western medicine in Europe in the nineteenth century. The newer synthetics replaced marijuana because of their dose reliability, ease of administration, and decreased adverse effects. In 1937 the United States Congress enacted the Marijuana Tax Act, which declared marijuana use illegal.[46]

In the drug culture of the 1960's, marijuana again increased in popularity. In 1982 the NIDA high school survey reported that 6.3 per cent of high school seniors are daily users of marijuana. NIDA's household survey reports that the daily use among young adults (18 to 25 years) is 21 per cent for some months during their life.[2]

In a 1975 survey, Corder et al. found that athletes used marijuana with the same incidence as nonathletes. This contrasted with the findings of a 1970 survey that found less use among athletes, dispelling the myth that sports "protect" the participant from chemical use.[47]

Some believe marijuana is a benign drug that should be legalized or at least that the laws should be changed to take a more lenient stance against the marijuana user. This has been done in a number of locations. Others still maintain that marijuana laws should not be loosened and that the effects of the drug necessitate its continued treatment as a dangerous drug. Between these two extremes lie many varied opinions about marijuana. It is hoped that one would educate oneself prior to taking a position on the continuum of opinions regarding this drug.

PHARMACOLOGY

Marijuana is derived from the leaves of the *Cannabis sativa* hemp plant. Easily cultivated, it has been grown in fields, plant boxes, and basements. Tetrahydrocannabinol (THC) is the active ingredient. THC is difficult to synthesize and, although reportedly sold in pill form in the street market, this pill form has been analyzed as another sedative drug (phencyclidine) in most cases.[1]

The lipid-soluble THC is absorbed rapidly when smoked but has a short-term effect. The half-life of THC is approximately five days, but owing to its lipid solubility and storage, the removal of the majority of THC can take a month.[48]

The mechanism of action of marijuana is similar to that of alcohol and the barbiturates—diffuse depression of the central nervous system.[1]

As with all sedative-hypnotic drugs, marijuana relieves anxiety, can produce ataxia, sedation, anesthesia, excitement, disinhibition, drunkenness, and respiratory and vasomotor depression. These effects are dose-related. Habituation is seen with increasing use.[1]

Some effects that have been noted with THC use include:

1. Decreases in intraocular pressure.[49–51] Others have shown no change in intraocular pressure.[52, 53] When found, this effect lasts for several hours.[46]

2. Bronchodilation lasting a period that paralleled the high blood level of THC.[46, 54, 55]

3. Increased appetite.[48]

Therapeutically there have been trials of marijuana in an attempt to treat asthmatics, glaucoma patients, and cancer patients during chemotherapy. There has not been widespread acceptance for the same reasons that the use of marijuana was curtailed earlier this century—dose unreliability, difficulty of administration, and decreased adverse effects of other available medications.[46]

EFFECTS ON PERFORMANCE

For athletic performance to be consistently successful, optimal physical, mental, and emotional states are necessary. The effects of marijuana on the perceptions of the user would make it difficult for him to perform optimally. Perception of time is altered, which usually results in a slow-motion effect. Depth perception, which is important in all games involving a ball and other activities, is decreased. There is an impairment of immediate memory which is critical in events that require strategies and teamwork. Other effects that can be noted during acute intoxication with marijuana include enhanced imagery, distortion of space and time, euphoria and relaxation, impairment of recent memory, increased suggestibility and sometimes depersonalization, suspiciousness, and panic reactions.[48] All of these effects make it difficult for the athlete to perform.

O'Brien describes the amotivational syndrome, which includes apathy, unwillingness or inability to carry out tasks to completion, low threshold of frustration, unrealistic thinking, increased introversion, and total involvement in the present at the expense of future goals. This is refuted by some studies while still maintained as a factor by others.[48]

Physiologically an increase has been shown in heart rate response to exercise with a diminished duration of exercise.[46, 56]

ADVERSE EFFECTS

The perceptual and behavioral changes were described in the previous section. Other areas that are adversely affected by the use of marijuana include:

1. Weakening of the bronchial defenses against infection through changes in the alveolar macrophages.[46, 56, 57]
2. Atrophy of certain areas of the brain with long-term use.[59]
3. In some animal species, an increase in spontaneous abortions and stillbirths.[48]

The psychological and behavioral effects are the most dangerous, especially if one considers high-risk situations such as driving or operating heavy machinery. The changes in perception and subsequent judgments that are dependent upon those perceptions can magnify the already large problem of chemical-related accidents, both motor vehicle and work-related.

SUMMARY

Marijuana is a sedative-hypnotic that is derived from the leaf of the *Cannabis sativa* plant. The actions of marijuana are similar to those of alcohol and the other drugs of this class. Marijuana has been shown to adversely affect a number of systems, including the pulmonary and nervous systems. No positive benefit has been shown from the use of marijuana by athletes.

SEDATIVES

HISTORY

Since the early twentieth century, a class of drugs known as sedatives has been utilized to relieve anxiety and induce sleep. These drugs have a high abuse potential owing to their ability to relieve stress and the willingness of many to use pharmacology to deal with the unwanted and bothersome stresses of life. The escape afforded by these drugs is temporary, and if the causes of stress remain unchanged, dependence on the drug becomes a possibility.

The National Institute of Drug Abuse in its 1982 survey reported that 14.9 per cent of youth (12 to 17 years), 29 per cent of young adults (18 to 25 years), and 62.7 per cent of older adults (26 years and over) have had a prescription for a sedative or tranquilizer. Nonmedical daily use of sedatives occurs among only 0.5 per cent of high school seniors. However 10.7 per cent of youth, 33.8 per cent of young adults, and 8.4 per cent of older adults reported nonmedical use of these medications.[2]

PHARMACOLOGY

The sedative class of drugs includes:

1. Monoureides (e.g., carbromal)
2. Barbiturates (e.g., pentobarbital [Nembutal])
3. Piperidinedione derivatives (e.g., glutethimide [Doriden])
4. Carbamates and dicarbamates (e.g., methocarbamol [Robaxin])
5. Benzodiazepines (e.g., diazepam [Valium])

The action of these drugs is depression of the central nervous system. Their effects include sedation, disinhibition, relief of anxiety, sleep, anesthesia, analgesia, anticonvulsant action, and voluntary muscle relaxation. These effects explain the clinical use of these drugs for sleep induction, muscle relaxation, and anxiety relief (e.g., in preoperative medication).

EFFECTS ON PERFORMANCE

As with all "downers," the reason for use by athletes is to decrease anxiety and deal with the stress of competition or with the stresses of life in general that are affecting performance.

Studies have shown that performance while using a sedative is diminished, but the performance was perceived by the athlete as being good.[60] As was the case with marijuana, the adverse effects of drowsiness, impaired judgment, impaired psychomotor performance, and hangover can lead to decreased physical and mental performance.[1, 60, 61]

ADVERSE EFFECTS

Many of the adverse effects described for alcohol and marijuana also are seen with sedatives, e.g., ataxia, nystagmus, withdrawal problems, dependency, and cardiovascular and respiratory depression. Also, the above-mentioned problems of drowsiness and impaired psychomotor skills further weigh on the negative side of the risk-benefit scale, which should be tallied prior to using any drug.

Overdosage with these drugs is a real problem. Both intentional and accidental suicides have been reported with the individual drugs or combinations of sedatives. One of the most dangerous combinations is the sedative and alcohol, which has resulted in death in a number of cases.

It is important to reiterate the hazard that is present for the individual and everyone around him or her if these drugs are taken while operating a motor vehicle or heavy machinery.

SUMMARY

Sedatives comprise a large class of drugs utilized both for therapy and as an escape ticket from the stresses of life. They have been shown to impair performance and have a number of adverse and potentially hazardous effects.

BETA-ADRENERGIC BLOCKERS

HISTORY

Propranolol (Inderal) was the first marketed beta-adrenergic blocking drug. The initial indication for propranolol was the treatment of angina pectoris. Other therapeutic uses for the beta blockers included cardiac arrhythmia, hypertension, pheochromocytoma, asymmetric septal hypertrophy (idiopathic hypertrophic subaortic stenosis), dissecting aortic aneurysm, thyrotoxicosis, anxiety states, migraine headaches, schizophrenia, and drug withdrawal syndromes. This is not an exhaustive list of the therapeutic indications for which trials were performed.

Athletes in sports requiring full control (archery, pistol and rifle shooting) as well as those athletes who have difficulty controlling anxiety have used beta blockers to attain their goals.

PHARMACOLOGY

The stimulation of the beta-adrenergic receptors results in vasodilation, cardiac stimulation, relaxation of nonvascular smooth muscle of the gut and bronchioles, and stimulation of glycolysis and lipolysis.[1, 3, 62] Beta-blockade has been divided into beta-1 and beta-2 receptor blockade. Beta-1 receptors are found in the heart, kidneys, and adipose tissue; beta-2 receptors are found in the liver, bronchi, and arteries.[63]

TABLE 7–2. Pharmacological Properties of Beta Blockers

Drug	Potency*	MSA	ISA	Cardioselectivity	Approved for Use in†
Atenolol (Tenormin)	1	–	–	+	H
Metoprolol (Lopressor)	0.5–2	–	–	+	H, AMI
Nadolol (Corgard)	0.5–4	–	–	–	H, A
Pindolol (Visken)	5–10	+	+	–	H
Propranolol (Inderal)	1	+	–	–	H, A, IHSS, M, Arr, P, PMI
(Inderal-LA)	1	+	–	–	H, A, IHSS, M
Timolol (Blocadren)	5–10	–	–	–	H, PMI

*Relative to propranolol
†MSA = Membrane-stabilizing activity
 ISA = Intrinsic sympathomimetic activity
   H = Hypertension
 AMI = Acute myocardial infarction
   A = Angina
IHSS = Idiopathic hypertrophic subaortic stenosis
   M = Migraine
 Arr = Arrhythmia
   P = Pheochromocytoma
 PMI = Postmyocardial infarction
Adapted from Moses JW: Beta-adrenergic blocking agents. Primary Cardiol 1(Suppl):138, 1984.

Theoretically, a beta-1 blocking agent would have an effect on heart rate and lipolysis but no effect on bronchospasm and glycogenolysis. However, it has been found that with higher doses of beta-1 blockers, beta-2 blockade becomes evident.[62]

The pharmacological properties of the available beta blockers vary, and these are presented in Tables 7–2 and 7–3.

It is important to be familiar with the properties of the various drugs prior to matching a patient with a particular drug. Propranolol is approved for use in the treatment of migraine headaches. It is the only beta blocker with high lipophilic ratings (lipid soluble).

Another important factor when dealing with athletes is the effect of a drug on energy production via lipolysis and glycogenolysis. Beta blockers affect both avenues of energy production and therefore may not be the optimal therapeutic tool in the athlete, especially one participating in endurance events.

EFFECTS ON PERFORMANCE

Two groups of people should be discussed in this section. The first is the individual who has a disease process that is limiting his or her activity, e.g., the individual with angina. The other is the individual with a normal cardiovascular system who takes the beta blocker for other reasons, such as migraines, anxiety, or essential tremor.

With cardiovascular disease, studies have shown that the positive effects of exercise training were unchanged by the chronic use of beta blockers.[64-67] No differences were noted using various types of beta blockers. These studies show that the individual who has cardiovascular disease can receive the same benefits from an exercise program whether or not beta blocker therapy is used.

The acute response to exercise while using beta blockers has shown results that vary from decreases in maximum oxygen uptake[68] to no change[69] to increases.[70] Many factors have been suggested to explain these different findings, including the timing of test and last dose,

TABLE 7–3. Pharmacokinetic Properties of Beta Blockers

	Average Serum Half-Life (h)	Elimination	Systemic Availability* (%)	Total Daily Dose	Acute IV Dose (mg)
Atenolol	7	R	55	50–200	5–10
Metoprolol	4	H	50	50–450	10–15
Nadolol	18	R	20	40–560	—
Pindolol	3.5	H-R	90	2.5–30	0.4–2
Propranolol	4.5	H	33	40–960	1–15
Timolol	4.5	H	75	15–60	0.4–1

*Combining gastrointestinal absorption and first-pass metabolism.
R = Renal
H = Hepatic
Adapted from Moses JW: Beta-adrenergic blocking agents. Primary Cardiol (Suppl 1):138, 1984.

duration of time on medication, method of drug administration, dosage of drug, type of test (cycle vs. treadmill), protocol of exercise test, and population studies (healthy normals vs. diseased).[70]

When preparing an exercise program for an individual using beta blockers, it is suggested that the exercise test (cycle or treadmill) be performed while on the medication. The timing of medication dose and exercise test should be similar to the timing of medication dose and exercise during training.[70] The use of perceived exertion is difficult in the patient using beta-blockers, since these drugs have been shown to alter the correlation between perceived exertion and heart rate.[72]

The effect of beta blockers on anxiety and essential tremor forms the rationale for their use by certain athletes. Beta blockers have been shown to improve performance in musicians.[71] Athletes who require steadiness can benefit from the calming effects of these drugs. Included in this group are the shooters and archers. The potential adverse effects of these drugs deter other athletes from using them.

ADVERSE EFFECTS

All drugs have adverse effects and the beta blockers are no exception. The more beta-1 selective the drug, the fewer adverse effects are seen.[70]

Bronchospasm can result, especially in individuals who have a history of asthma. Untoward cardiovascular effects include hypotension, congestive heart failure, bradycardia, and atrioventricular block. Peripherally, vasoconstriction can occur as well as Raynaud's phenomenon. With the lipophilic drugs, central nervous system disturbances and hallucinations or vivid dreams have been reported. Hypoglycemia can be seen, and this effect is easily understood in view of the effect on glycogenolysis. Impotence has been reported by some males taking these drugs. Other general effects include gastrointestinal disturbance and reversible alopecia.[63] Gradual withdrawal has been suggested when discontinuing the use of beta blockers to avoid worsening of symptoms of angina, palpitations, tremor, tachycardia, sweating, anxiety, or headaches.[72]

Adverse effects vary with the different drugs found among the beta blockers. They also can be related to the dosage, duration, and frequency of drug administration.

SUMMARY

Beta blockers have been useful in the treatment of angina, hypertension, arrhythmias, anxiety, and migraine headaches. The effects on the beta-adrenergic system have been separated into beta-1, which includes the heart, adipose tissue, and kidneys, and beta-2, which includes the liver, arteries, and bronchi. Therapeutically, beta blockers are used most commonly for cardiac-related problems, which have popularized the beta-1 blockers. Exercise training in the individual with cardiovascular problems is not affected by the chronic use of beta blockers. There is disagreement about acute use and the effect on exercise. Athletes use beta blockers to decrease anxiety and essential tremor. They are reported to be banned for the 1988 Olympic Games. Adverse effects include bronchospasm, hypotension, congestive heart failure, impotence, and CNS disturbances. When prescribing beta blockers to a competitive athlete, one must consider all factors and perhaps search for a better alternative.

REFERENCES

1. Meyers FH, Jawetz E, Goldfien A: Review of Medical Pharmacology, 6th ed. Los Altos, CA, Lange Publications, 1978.
2. National Institute on Drug Abuse. National Survey on Drug Abuse: Main Findings, 1982. U.S. Department of Health and Human Services. Public Health Service. Alcohol, Drug Abuse and Mental Health Administration, Rockville, MD, DHHS Publication No. (ADM), pp 83–1263, 1983.
3. Crossland J: Lewis' Pharmacology. 5th ed. New York, Churchill Livingstone, 1980.
4. Goldfrank L, Bresnitz E, Melinek M, et al: Antabuse. Hosp Phys 12:34–39, 1980.
5. Coopersmith S: The effects of alcohol on reaction to affective stimuli. Q J Stud Alcohol 25:459–475, 1964.
6. Huntley M: Effects of alcohol, uncertainty and novelty upon response selection. Psychopharmacologia 39:259–266, 1974.
7. Huntley M: Influences of alcohol and S-R uncertainty upon spatial localization time. Psychopharmacologia 27:131–140, 1972.
8. Nelson D: Effects of ethyl alcohol on the performance of selected gross motor tests. Res Q 30:312–320, 1959.
9. Moskowitz H, Burns M: Effect of alcohol on the psychological refractory period. Q J Stud Alcohol 32:782–790, 1971.
10. Carpenter J: Effects of alcohol on some psychological processes. Q J Stud Alcohol 23:274–314, 1962.
11. Collins W, Schroeder D, Gibson R, et al: Effects of alcohol ingestion on tracking performance during angular acceleration. J Appl Psychol 55:559–563, 1971.
12. Forney R, Hughes F, Greatbatch W: Measurement of attentive motor performance after alcohol. Percept Mot Skills 19:151–154, 1964.
13. Rundell O, Williams H: Alcohol and speed accuracy trade-off. Hum Factors 21:433–443, 1979.
14. Begbie G: The effects of alcohol and of varying amounts of visual information on a balancing test. Ergonomics 9:325–333, 1966.
15. Belgrave B, Bird K, Chester G, et al: The effect of cannabidiol, alone and in combination with ethanol, on human performance. Psychopharmacology 64:243–246, 1979.
16. Tang P, Rosenstein R: Influence of alcohol and Dramamine alone and in combination on psychomotor performance. Aerospace Med 39:818–821, 1967.
17. Enger N, Simonson E, Ballard G: The effect of small doses of alcohol in the central nervous system. Am J Clin Pathol 14:333–341, 1944.
18. Hebbellinck M: The effects of a moderate dose of alcohol on a series of functions of physical performance in man. Acta Int Pharmacol 120:402–405, 1959.
19. Hebbellinck M: The effects of a small dose of ethyl alcohol on certain basic components of human physical performance. Arch Int Pharmacodyn Ther 143:247–257, 1963.
20. Williams MH: Effect of selected doses of alcohol on fatigue parameters of the forearm flexor muscles. Res Q 40:832–840, 1969.
21. Phikanen T: Neurological and physiological studies on distilled and brewed beverages. Ann Med Exp Biol Fenn 35(Suppl 9):1–152, 1957.
22. Bobo W: Effects of alcohol upon maximum oxygen uptake, lung ventilation and heart rate. Res Q 43:1–6, 1972.
23. Mazers R, Picon-Reategive E, Thomas R: Effects of alcohol and altitude on man during rest and work. Aerospace Med 39:403–406, 1968.
24. Williams MH: Effect of small and moderate doses of alcohol on exercise heart rate and oxygen consumption. Res Q 43:94–104, 1972.

25. Bond V, Franks BD, Hawley ET: Effects of small and moderate doses of alcohol on submaximal cardiorespiratory function, perceived exertion and endurance performance in abstainers and moderate drinkers. J Sports Med 23:221–228, 1983.
26. Blonqvist G, Saltin B, Mitchell J: Acute effects of ethanol ingestion on the response to submaximal and maximal exercise in man. Circulation 42:463–470, 1970.
27. Department of Health, Education and Welfare. Third special report to the U.S. Congress on alcohol and health. NIAAA Information and Feature Service. DHEW Publication No. (ADM) pp 78–151, November 30, 1978.
28. Friedman H: Alcohol and heart disease. Primary Cardiol. December 1984, pp 44–48.
29. Haskell WL, Camargo C, Williams PT, et al: The effects of cessation and resumption of moderate alcohol intake on serum high-density lipoprotein subfractions: A controlled study. N Engl J Med 310:805–810, 1984.
30. Mills JL, Graubard BI, Harley EE, et al: Maternal alcohol consumption and birth weight. How much drinking during pregnancy is safe? JAMA 252(14):1875–1880, 1984.
31. Jones KL, Smith DW, Ulleland CN, et al: Pattern of malformation in offspring of chronic alcoholic mothers. Lancet 1:1267–1271, 1973.
32. Strissgirth AP: Fetal alcohol syndrome. An epidemiologic perspective. Am J Epidemiol 107:467–478, 1978.
33. Wilson GT: The effects of alcohol on male and female sexual function. Sex Med Today December 1984, pp 6–15.
34. Smith JW: Alcohol: Its effect on sexual performance. Consultant May 1982, pp 261–264.
35. Jablecki C: Neurological complications of alcoholism. Cont Educ January 1982, pp 23–25.
36. American College of Sports Medicine: Position Statement on the Use of Alcohol in Sports. Med Sci Sports Exerc 14(6):9–11, 1982.
37. Eriksson A, Bjomstig U: Fatal snowmobile accidents in northern Sweden. J Trauma 22(12):977–982, 1982.
38. Giersten J: Drowning while under the influence of alcohol. Med Sci Law 10:216–219, 1970.
39. Dietz PE, Baker SP: Drowning: Epidemiology and prevention. Am J Public Health 64:303–312, 1974.
40. Plueckhahn VD: Alcohol consumption and death by drowning in adults. A 24 year epidemiological analysis. J Stud Alcohol 43(5):445–452, 1982.
41. Isselbacher KJ: Metabolic and hepatic effects of alcohol. N Engl J Med 296:612, 1977.
42. Becker CE: Medical consequences of alcohol abuse. Postgrad Med 64(6):88–93, December 1978.
43. Kissin B, Kaley MM, Su WH, et al: Head and neck cancer in alcoholics. JAMA 224:1174–1175, 1973.
44. Graham T, Dalton J: Effect of alcohol on man's response to mild activity in a cold environment. Aviat Space Environ Med 51 (8):793–796, 1980.
45. Ewing JA: Detecting alcoholism. The CAGE questionnaire. JAMA 252(4):1905–1907, 1984.
46. Tashkin DP, Soares JR, Hepler RS, et al: UCLA conference cannabis 1977. Ann Int Med 89:539–548, 1978.
47. Corder BW, Dezelsky TL, Toohey JV, et al: Trends in drug use behavior at ten Central Arizona high schools. Ariz Health Recreat 19(1): Fall 1975.
48. O'Brien JE: Marijuana: New concerns versus possible new uses. Consultant, Fall 1982, pp 306–321.
49. Shapiro D: The ocular manifestation of the cannabinols. Ophthalmologica 168:366–369, 1974.
50. Purnell WD, Gregg JM: Delta 9 tetrahydrocannabinol, euphoria and intraocular pressure in man. Ann Ophthalmol 7:921–923, 1975.
51. Hepler RS, Frank IM, Petrus R: Ocular effects of marijuana smoking. In Braude MC, Szara S (eds): The Pharmacology of Marihuana, Vol 2. New York, Raven Press, 1976, p 815.
52. Flom MC, Adams AJ, Jones RT: Marijuana smoking and reduced pressure in human eyes: Drug action or epiphenomenon. Invest Ophthalmol Vis Sci 14:52–55, 1975.
53. Green K, Bowman K: Effect of marijuana and derivatives on aqueous human dynamics

in the rabbit. In Braude MC, Szara S (eds): The Pharmacology of Marihuana, Vol 2. New York, Raven Press, 1976, p 803.

54. Lemberger L, Axelrod J, Kopin IJ: Metabolism and disposition of delta-9-tetrahydrocannabinol in man. Pharm Rev 23:371–380, 1971.

55. Vachon L, Fitzgerald M, Solliday NH, et al: Single dose effect of marijuana smoke: Bronchial dynamics and respiratory center sensitivity in normal subjects. N Engl J Med 288:985–989, 1973.

56. Shapiro BJ, Reiss S, Sullivan SF, et al: Cardiopulmonary effects of marijuana smoking during exercise (abstract). Chest 70:441, 1976.

57. Mann PEG, Cohen AB, Finley TN, et al: Alveolar macrophage: Structural and functional differences between non-smokers and smokers of marijuana and tobacco. Lab Invest 25:111–120, 1971.

58. Huber GL, Simmons GA, McCarthy CR, et al: Depressant effect of marijuana smoke on antibactericidal activity of pulmonary alveolar macrophages. Chest 68:769–773, 1975.

59. McGahon JP, Dublin AB, Sassenroth E: Long term delta 9 tetrahydrocannabinol treatment: Computed tomography of the brains of rhesus monkeys. Am J Dis Child 138:1109–1112, 1984.

60. Smith GM, Beecher HK: Amphetamines, secobarbital and athletic performance. III. Quantitative effects on judgment. JAMA 172(15):1623–1629, 1960.

61. Blum B, Stern MH, Melville KI: A comparative evaluation of the actions of depressant and stimulant drugs on human performance. Psychopharmacology 6:171–177, 1964.

62. Allen CJ, et al: Beta blockade and exercise in normal subjects and patients with coronary artery disease. Phys Sports Med 12(10):51–63, 1984.

63. Moses JW: Beta adrenergic blocking agents. Primary Cardiol (Suppl 1): 137–143, 1984.

64. Dressendorfer R, Smith MA, Gordon S, et al: Improved maximal oxygen uptake during phase 2 cardiac rehabilitation is independent of beta-blockade therapy (abstract). J Am Coll Cardiol 3:500, 1984.

65. Laslett L, et al: Exercise training efficacy is not affected by propranolol administration in coronary patients (abstract). Am J Cardiol 50:1070, 1982.

66. Vanhees L, Fagard R, Amery A: Influence of beta-adrenergic blockade on the hemodynamic effects of physical training in patients with ischemic heart disease. Am Heart J 108:270–275, 1984.

67. Fletcher GF: Exercise training during chronic beta blockade in cardiovascular disease. Am J Cardiol 55:1100–1130, 1985.

68. Wilmore JH, Ewy GA, Morton AR, et al: The effect of beta-adrenergic blockade on submaximal and maximal exercise performance. J Cardiac Rehabil 3:30–36, 1983.

69. Sklar J, Johnston GD, Overlie P, et al: The effects of a cardioselective (metoprolol) and a non-selective (propranolol) beta-adrenergic blocker in the response to dynamic exercise in normal men. Circulation 65:894–899, 1982.

70. Wilmore JH, Freund BJ, Joyner MJ, et al. Acute response to submaximal and maximal exercise consequent to beta-adrenergic blockade: Implications for the prescription of exercise. Am J Cardiol 55:135D–141D, 1985.

71. Brantigan CO, Brantigan TA, Joseph N: Effect of beta-blockade and beta-stimulation on stage fright. Am J Med 72:88–94, 1982.

72. Nattel S: Prevention of beta-blocker withdrawal syndromes. Primary Cardiol (Hosp Phys Suppl): 37–39, 1981.

8

DETECTION OF DRUG USE BY ATHLETES

DON H. CATLIN, M.D.

The term "doping" may have originated from "dop," a South African drink composed of cola nut extracts, alcohol, and xanthines.[1] Dictionaries categorize dope or doping as slang; nevertheless, the term is widely used even in formal publications. The European Council defined doping as "the administering or use of substances in any form alien to the body or of physiological substances in abnormal amounts and with abnormal methods by healthy persons with the exclusive aim of attaining an artificial and unfair increase of performance in competition."[2] This is a satisfactory and certainly convenient definition in the present context. Understanding doping control requires synthesizing knowledge drawn from clinical sciences, pharmacology, and analytical chemistry. Applying the principles and practice of analytical chemistry establishes whether or not a drug or metabolite is present and, in some cases, the quantity of drug in a body fluid. Interpretation of the findings utilizes clinical, statistical, and pharmacologic principles, particularly those related to decision analysis, pharmacokinetics, and metabolism. This chapter focuses on analytical methods used to detect banned agents from a general perspective in the context of providing analytical support for international competition.

BACKGROUND

The impetus for developing doping control laboratories began in the late 1950's and 1960's with reports of widespread misuse of drugs in the athletic community. At the Rome Olympics in 1960, a Danish cyclist died under the influence of stimulants, and in 1967 a Tour de France contestant succumbed to the influence of amphetamine.[3-5] Questionnaires administered at the 1964 games in Tokyo evidently revealed a high incidence of drug misuse that prompted Olympic physicians to demand action.[5] Confronted with reports of stimulant abuse among cyclists, Belgium and France passed anti-doping laws in 1965. The International Cycling Federation was the first international organization to introduce doping control rules. Now all federations prohibit doping. The International Olympic Committee (IOC) responded by establishing a Medical Commission (MC) in 1967 under the chairmanship of Prince de Merode of Belgium and listed doping control as a major responsibility of the commission.[5] Today the recommendations and regulations of the IOC/ MC play a major role in doping control and, in particular, in the development and accreditation of doping control laboratories.

Urged by the International Cycling Federation, laboratories in Europe began testing in the early 1960's, but the tests appeared to be insensitive because continued drug use was not detected.[3] In 1965 sensitive gas chromatography (GC) techniques were introduced by Beckett [3,6] for the Tour of Britain race with results that included the disqualification of three individuals. The IOC conducted preliminary testing for the 1968 games, but it was not until the 1972 summer games in Munich that comprehensive testing was conducted at a major international event.[7-10]

GC combined with mass spectrometry (MS) is the most sensitive, rigorous, and specific analytical technique that is practical for doping control. Since 1972, the IOC and virtually all international sports federations have required GC/MS identification of the drugs or metabolites for all positive cases. This requirement, together with the lack of a satisfactory screening technique, delayed the introduction of effective testing for anabolic steroids until 1976. It was well known that anabolic steroids were being used in the 1960's, but it was not until Brooks developed radioimmunoassays (RIA) for anabolic steroids[11, 12] that it became practical to screen a large number of samples over a short period of time. The RIA, together with developments in the field of GC/MS methods for anabolic steroids, enabled the IOC to add anabolic steroids to their list of banned substances for the 1976 Montreal games.[7, 13, 14] For the 1984 Olympic Games in Los Angeles, the UCLA laboratory performed a GC/ MS analysis for anabolic steroids on all 1500 samples. This effort was facilitated by a combination of reliable instruments equipped with autosamplers, a powerful computer, advice from previous Olympic laboratories, and a dedicated and experienced staff.

DOPING AGENTS AND CLASSES

One aspect of the work of the IOC/MC is publication of a Medical Controls Brochure in conjunction with each of the Olympic Games. The Brochure, which is a bylaw to Rule 29 of the Olympic Charter, contains doping regulations and a list of doping agents. The list from the 1984 Brochure is reproduced in Table 8–1. In May of 1985 the IOC/MC added

TABLE 8–1. Substances Banned by the International Olympic Committee at the 1984 Summer Olympic Games—Doping Classes with Examples

A. Psychomotor stimulant drugs, e.g.:
amphetamine
benzphetamine
chlorphentermine
cocaine
diethylpropion
dimethylamphetamine
ethylamphetamine
fencamfamin
meclofenoxate
methylamphetamine
methylphenidate
norpseudoephedrine
pemoline
phendimetrazine
phenmetrazine
phentermine
pipradol
prolintane
   and related compounds

B. Sympathomimetic amines, e.g.:
chlorprenaline
ephedrine
etafedrine
isoetharine
isoprenaline
methoxyphenamine
methylephedrine
   and related compounds

C. Miscellaneous central nervous system stimulants, e.g.:
amiphenazole
bemigride
caffeine*
cropropamide (component of "micoren")
crotethamide (component of "micoren")
doxapram
ethamivan
leptazol
nikethamide
picrotoxine
strychnine
   and related compounds

D. Narcotic analgesics, e.g.:
anileridine
codeine
dextromoramide
dihydrocodeine
dipipanone
ethylmorphine
heroin
hydrocodone
hydromorphone
levorphanol
methadone
morphine
oxomorphone
pentazocine
pethidine
phenazocine
piminodine
thebacon
trimeperidine
   and related compounds

E. Anabolic steroids, e.g.:
clostebol
dehydrochlormethyltestosterone
fluoxymesterone
mesterolone
methenolone
methandienone
methyltestosterone
nandrolone
norethandrolone
oxymesterone
oxymetholone
stanozolol
testosterone*
   and related compounds

P.S. At the request of the International Federations concerned (F.I.E. and U.I.P.M.B.) an alcohol test will be carried out during their competitions.

   *Definition of positive depends on the following:

For caffeine—if the concentration in urine exceeds 15 micrograms/ml

For testosterone—if the ratio of the total concentration of testosterone to that of epitestosterone in the urine exceeds 6.

blood doping and beta blockers to the list.[15] In the latter case, the ban is limited to those International Sports Federations that specifically ban beta blockers, for example, the Union Internationale de Pentathlon Moderne et Biathlon (UIPMB).

DRUG METABOLISM CONSIDERATIONS

Most drugs are metabolized to one or more metabolites before they are excreted, and some are almost completely metabolized. For example, after a dose of methylphenidate (Ritalin) or cocaine, the urine contains ritalinic acid or benzoylecgonine, respectively.[16, 17] After the oral administration of methandienone (Dianabol), the urine contains 6α-hydroxy-17-epi-methandienone and 17-epi-methandienone, but not methandienone itself.[18] These two metabolites of methandienone are found "free" in the urine. In contrast, some anabolic steroids become conjugated to a glucose or sulfate group in the body; thus, a deconjugation step (usually with β-glucuronidase or Helix pomatia preparation) is a prerequisite to recovering all the available drug. The ratio of metabolite to the parent compound may exceed 10:1, and the concentration of the parent drug may be low. Therefore, the detection of these substances often depends on finding the metabolites.

The degree to which the metabolism of individual doping agents has been investigated in man is quite variable. The scientific literature contains many papers on the human metabolism of amphetamine, cocaine, morphine, and other drugs listed in Table 8–1, but there is much less published literature on others, particularly some of the anabolic steroids. In the latter situation, it may be necessary to conduct clinical trials to obtain the reference analytical data. In the case of drugs that are not approved by the U.S. Food and Drug Administration or of veterinary compounds, animal studies or clinical samples donated by individuals who take the drugs of their own accord may be utilized.

PERIOD OF DETECTABILITY

How long after discontinuing drugs can they still be detected? This is the most commonly asked question, but it defies a simple answer because of the large number of variables that affect the answer and the limited amount of published data. The principal determinants are dose; drug formulation; route of administration; body burden of drug at the time of discontinuation; pharmacokinetic factors; clinical factors such as renal function, body composition, and hydration; and analytical factors such as the detection limit of the assay and the volume of the sample.

The discussion is simplified by considering the drugs in groups A through D of Table 8–1 as one large group, which may be referred to as nonanabolic drugs or as the stimulants and opioids. Group E, the anabolic steroids, is a second large group. Virtually all drugs listed in Table 8–1 are readily detected for several hours (in many cases days) after drug administration. However, the purpose and pattern of use must be considered when interpreting testing results. Except for anabolic steroids, all drugs in Table 8–1 may be considered to have the potential to enhance performance only if they are taken just before a competitive event. Since the samples are collected within a few hours of the event—that is, at the time when the urine usually contains a large amount of drug, virtually all drug use is detected. Accordingly, testing is an effective deterrent to stimulant-enhanced performance.

Anabolic steroids may be considered training drugs, that is, drugs taken during the training period for the purpose of enhancing performance at a future event. There is no evidence that acute single doses enhance performance. Clearly, if anabolic steroids are discontinued before the event in sufficient time to permit the urinary concentration of drug to fall below the detection limit of the assay (about 1 to 10 ng/ml), the test will be negative. The only published data that pertain to this issue utilized subjects who received a single dose of steroids. For example, the metabolites of nandrolone are detectable for about 50 days after a 25-mg parenteral dose,[19] and methandrostenolone is detectable for 4 days after a 10-mg oral dose.[20] What is known about the kinetics of steroids suggests that large doses consumed over many days will establish substantial body burdens and prolong excretion of drugs and metabolites. Anecdotal reports of detection times of several months are probably not exaggerated in the case of nandrolone and other steroids formulated in oil. I have interviewed some users who give such histories, but I can never be certain if the history is accurate, and the user may not know pertinent dosage details. Detection times for 17-alkylated anabolic steroids are much shorter (days to weeks) and appear to be highly variable.

GENERAL METHODS OF DETECTION

From the analytical perspective, the task is to develop methods for detecting all the drugs or the metabolites of the drugs listed in Table 8–1 and as many of the related substances as is practical. This is accomplished by an integrated sequence of procedures and methods that includes (1) sample preparation, (2) performing several screening procedures on each sample, and (3) performing confirmation or identification procedures on those samples that are not declared negative after reviewing the results of the screening procedures.

First, the sample is split into several aliquots, one for each screening procedure. Depending on the particular screening procedure, the preparation steps include extraction, hydrolysis (which includes deconjugation), and derivatization. The purposes of these chemical steps are to concentrate and partially purify the substances and to alter their chemical characteristics so that they will be suitable for analysis by the screening procedure. For example, analysis by GC requires volatilization of the substances, yet many are not particularly volatile; therefore, a derivatization step is included to transform them into volatile products. Following the preparation step, the extracts are analyzed by several different techniques such as GC, liquid chromatography, immunoassay, and GC/MS. When these methods are used to screen large numbers of samples, the analysis is designed to search for as many drugs as is practical, and the method is referred to as a screening procedure. After completing the screening procedures, the samples are divided into two categories, a negative group and a group that requires further analysis. In the latter case, the data from the screening procedure indicate that a doping agent and/or metabolites may be present; additionally, the screen usually provides preliminary identification of the agents.

The confirmation step provides unequivocal identification of the drug and/or metabolites. As previously noted, IOC regulations require analysis and identification of all positive cases by GC/MS. This is a stringent requirement and differs from other situations that clinicians may be more familiar with. In the case of athletics, false-positive results are not tolerable, thereby justifying the use of expensive and sophisticated confirmation procedures. In the case of routine clinical toxicology, false positive results are also undesirable, but the data show that mistakes do occur.[22, 23]

CHROMATOGRAPHY

Chromatography is a method of separating components of a mixture by partitioning the components into two phases, one stationary and the other mobile.[24] The sample containing the substances to be separated is introduced into the mobile phase, which may be a gas or liquid. The stationary phase may be paper (paper chromatography), a glass plate coated with a thin layer of fine granular powder (thin layer chromatography), granular powder contained in a column (column chromatography), or a liquid or solid immobilized in a column (gas chromatography). As the mobile phase (solvent) moves past the stationary phase, the components of the mixture repeatedly partition between the two phases, resulting in some substances being retarded more than others. The partitioning process is based on physical characteristics of the molecules. In the case of column chromatography, the first portions of the mobile phase to emerge from the column (eluate) contain the substances that are least retarded by the stationary phase; later eluates contain substances that interact to a greater degree with the column. Figure 8–1 shows two substances that are not completely resolved by the chromatographic process (left pair) and two substances that are well separated (right pair). The retention times (RT) of substances 1 and 2 are $t_1 = 15.40$ and $t_2 = 15.65$, respectively.

Many different types of chromatography are available, for example, paper and thin layer,[25] liquid and liquid solid,[26] and gas liquid and gas solid.[27] The most commonly used types of chromatography in doping control laboratories are liquid, thin layer, and gas chromatography.

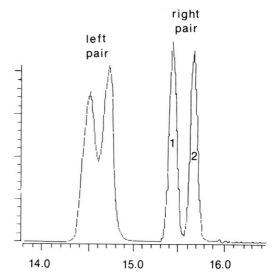

Figure 8–1. Chromatogram showing poor separation (left pair) and good separation (right pair) of two peaks.

THIN LAYER CHROMATOGRAPHY (TLC)

The stationary phase is prepared by applying a thin layer of solid support (e.g., silica gel) to the surface of a glass plate. The substances to be studied are "spotted" on the surface along a line marked as the origin (Fig. 8–2). The plate is placed upright in a chamber filled with the mobile phase to a depth just below the origin. As the mobile phase moves upward by capillary action, the compounds are carried upward to various degrees. The plate is removed when the front approaches the top of the plate, and the solvent front is marked. The location of colorless substances is determined by fluorescence under ultraviolet light, staining reactions, or a variety of other techniques. Compounds are characterized by calculating R_f values where

$$R_f = \frac{\text{distance travelled by substance X}}{\text{distance travelled by mobile phase}}$$

In Figure 8–2 the R_f for compound A is $75/100 = 0.75$. By comparing the R_f value for an unknown to R_f values for reference compounds, the analyst tentatively identifies the unknown.

As described above, TLC is a rapid, simple, and inexpensive technique, but it may lack accuracy. This problem is overcome by determining R_f values with a second (or more) system that utilizes different mobile or stationary phases or by detecting the "spot" by a different principle. Considering the multiplicity of factors that determine the accuracy of TLC, it is apparent that no summary statement would apply to all cases. An optimized TLC system is highly specific and accurate. Similarly, the

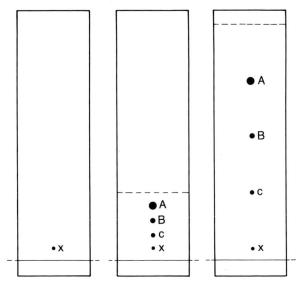

Figure 8–2. Illustration of three thin layer chromatography plates showing *(left)* the mixture to be separated spotted at the origin (X); *(middle)* after the solvent front (dashed line) has advanced and three spots (A, B, C) have separated from the origin; and *(right)* after the solvent front has nearly reached the edge of the plate and A, B, and C are fully separated.

detection limit or minimum amount of substance that can be detected (sensitivity, detection limit) with TLC is difficult to define without a detailed review of a system. In general, most of the drugs in Table 8–1 (groups A to D) can be identified by TLC with a detection limit of at least 1.0 μg/ml. Currently TLC is not practical for identifying anabolic steroids.

GAS CHROMATOGRAPHY[18]

Like TLC, there is no universally accepted procedure for performing gas chromatography (GC). There are innumerable types of columns, stationary phases, detectors, instruments, and methods of operating the instruments. Any given combination has advantages and disadvantages over other variations, and all can produce satisfactory results under the proper conditions. Figure 8–3 illustrates the principles of GC separation. A small volume of the final extract is taken up in a syringe and injected into a heated chamber positioned at the head of a column. The sample is immediately volatilized and swept into and eventually through the column by a carrier gas (mobile phase). While traversing the column, the compounds are repeatedly absorbed into and desorbed from the stationary phase. The substances are separated because they are more or less retarded in accordance with their individual partition rations between the two phases. The retention time (RT) or time of emergence of each substance from the column is reproducible and unique; therefore, the RT

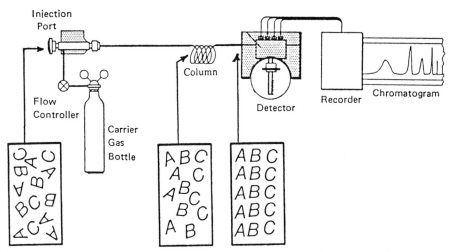

Figure 8–3. Schematic drawing of a gas chromatographic system and the process of separation. Immediately after injection, the drugs (A, B, C) are not separated *(left box)*. While traversing the column, the drugs begin to separate *(middle box)*, and they are completely separated by the time the sample strikes the detector *(right box)*. (Adapted in part from McNair HM, Bonelli EJ: Basic Gas Chromatography. Walnut Creek, CA, Varian Aerograph, 1968.)

of a substance is one of the most important means of identifying an unknown substance.[32] The presence of a substance is determined by a detector positioned at the end of the column. A recording device registers signals from the detector and displays the information as a graph of detector response versus time. The height and area of the peak correlate with the amount of substance present.

An important aspect of identification by GC is the nature or specificity of the detector. Many are available, but in doping control the most widely used are the flame ionization detector (FID), the nitrogen-phosphorus detector (NPD), and a mass spectrometer. The FID registers a peak if the substance, when burned, produces ions. Most organic substances produce such ions. The NPD responds to any substance that contains nitrogen or phosphorus, which is the case for all doping agents except anabolic steroids.

Figure 8–4 is a chromatogram resulting from the injection of a mixture of calibration standards into a gas chromatograph equipped with a nitrogen-phosphorus detector and a 6-foot-long, 2-mm internal diameter glass column packed with a granular powder coated with the liquid (stationary) phase. The components of the mixture were selected to include substances that would elute at various times over the entire chromatogram. Thus, pseudoephedrine-TFA (peak No. 1) with an RT of 1.42 minutes is the first substance to elute and strychnine (peak No. 10, RT = 14.94 min) is the last. Phenazine (peak No. 4) is not a doping agent. It is used here as an internal standard. This means that a small amount of phenazine is added to every sample at the beginning of the analysis, and one expects to find a peak with the RT of phenazine in every chromatogram. The appearance of this peak serves as a control for the chemical work-up procedure and a precise RT marker for the individual sample. Using the RT of phenazine as a reference point, the relative retention time (RRT) of any other peak is calculated by:

$$RRT = \frac{RT \text{ of unknown peak X}}{RT \text{ of internal standard (phenazine)}}$$

The RRT of a substance is a more reliable identifying characteristic than RT; thus RRT's are widely used and the principles have been described in detail.[28] In practice, the analyst determines RRT's of all the compounds of interest using pure reference standards. These are periodically checked with standard mixtures (Fig. 8–4), and unknowns are tentatively identified by comparing the RRT with a list of known RRT's. The RRT for the peak with an RT of 0.60 minute in Figure 8–5A is 0.12 (0.60/4.87 phenazine), which corresponds to the RRT for norephedrine-TFA (Fig. 8–5B). Subsequent analysis by GC/MS confirmed the presence of norephedrine in this sample. The finding of a peak with an RRT

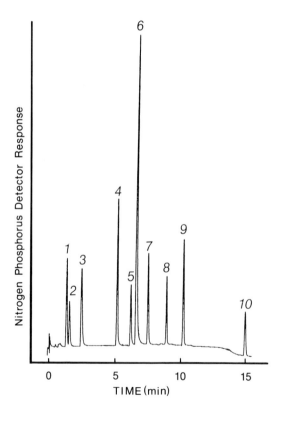

Figure 8–4. Gas chromatographic recording of a standard solution containing (1) pseudoephedrine-TFA, (2) *p*-hydroxyamphetamine-TFA, (3) *p*-hydroxymethamphetamine-TFA, (4) phenazine (internal standard), (5) levorphanol-TFA, (6) caffeine, (7) normethadone, (8) ethylmorphine-TFA, (9) hydrocodone, and (10) strychnine. (TFA = derivatized with trifluoroacetic acid anhydride.)

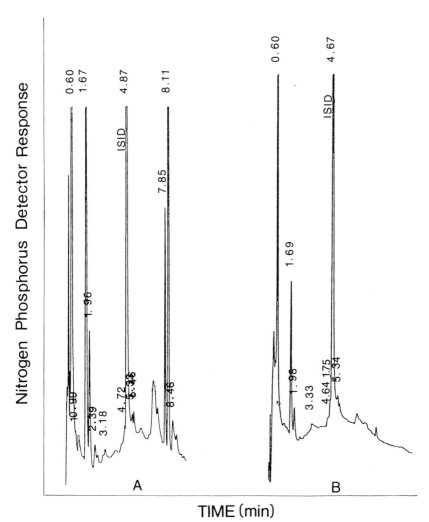

Figure 8–5. Gas chromatographic analysis of a urine sample obtained from an individual taking norephedrine *(A)* and from a blank urine spiked with norephedrine *(B)*. The figure demonstrates how gas chromatography may be used to identify a drug in an unknown urine. The chromatogram in *A* shows the internal standard (RT = 4.87 min) and several other peaks. The RRT of the peak with a RT of 0.60 min is 0.12, which corresponds to the RRT of norephedrine-TFA in the reference list. The result was checked by adding norephedrine to a blank urine *(B)*. The RT and RRT of the peak at 0.60 in *A* is identical to the RT and RRT of authentic norephedrine added to the sample in *B*, thus providing tentative identification of the peak as norephedrine-TFA.

identical to the RRT of a reference sample of pure drug does not prove that the peak is the drug because other substances may have the same RRT. If GC/MS is not available, the analyst could repeat the GC analysis on a different column. Many types of columns are available, and the RT and RRT of drugs vary from one type to another; therefore, the demonstration that a peak with the proper RRT for a drug occurs on two or more columns provides more conclusive evidence that the peak is the drug.

GAS CHROMATOGRAPHY/MASS SPECTROMETRY

When a mass spectrometer is used as a detector for a gas chromatograph, the combination is referred to as GC/MS. Like the other methods, there are many different types of mass spectrometers and many ways to perform mass spectrometry.[29] After exiting the GC column, the separated compounds enter the MS one by one. In the MS, under high vacuum, an electron beam ionizes each compound and/or cleaves it into ionized fragments. The MS uses a complex system of focusing devices and electrical force to resolve ions differing by one mass unit or less and propel them to a detector that measures the abundance of each ion. A given compound always breaks into the same fragment ions, so that a graph of the relative abundance of the ions (Y-axis) versus their mass (X-axis), or mass spectrum (Fig. 8–6C), virtually identifies the compound. The mass spectrum together with the RRT constitutes a most rigorous identification of a compound. A complete mass spectrum of the GC eluate is recorded about every second; therefore a computer is used to store, collate, and display the large number of data generated by each sample. Three commonly used outputs of a GC/MS data system are total ion current (TIC), the selected ion current, and the full mass spectrum. The TIC (Fig. 8–6A) consists of the sum of all the registered ions of all masses, each of which (at each mass) may be individually displayed in the selected ion current plot (Fig. 8–6B).

In practice, one develops a computer-based registry consisting of the RT, RRT, and spectrum of a large number of compounds collected under specific chemical and instrumental conditions. Identification of an unknown consists of finding a peak in the unknown that has the same RRT and spectrum as that of a known standard in the reference library. The literature contains many reviews of GC/MS techniques pertaining to steroids in general,[30, 31] anabolic steroids in the context of doping control,[32, 33] and nonanabolic steroids.[34]

IMMUNOCHEMICAL ASSAYS

Immunochemical techniques[35, 36] are widely applied in toxicology and clinical chemistry laboratories. Immunoassays are useful for screening large numbers of samples rapidly and inexpensively. However, cross-reactions between the antibodies and closely related endogenous or exogenous substances dictate that positive results be confirmed by other methods. Of the 56 drugs that comprise groups A through D of Table 8–1, commercial kits are available for only 5 or 6. Therefore, this technology has limited applicability to doping control for these groups. Brooks[11, 12] and others [37, 38] have investigated the problem of preparing antisera

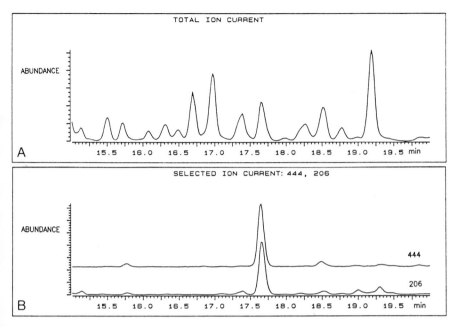

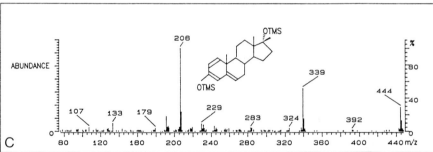

Figure 8–6. Examples of gas chromatography/mass spectrometry data. The total ion current *(A)* is the sum of the abundance of all ions monitored during the run. In this case 20 ions were monitored, including two (444,206) known to be present in the spectrum *(C)* of derivatized (di-TMS) epi-methandienone (epidianabol), a metabolite of methandienone. The predicted RT of epi-methandienone is 17.65 min. The peak at 17.65 min in *A* is shown to contain ions 444 and 206 *(B)*. The spectrum of this peak is shown in *C*. It is identical to the spectrum of epi-methandienone (di-TMS derivative).

suitable for screening urine samples for anabolic steroids. The task is to prepare immunogens that will induce the formation of antibodies with specificity for a large number of chemically similar anabolic steroids (group specificity), while at the same time discriminating against endogenous androgens and other steroids that are similar in structure to anabolic steroids. The 17α-methylated steroids can be detected with an antiserum prepared against 17α-methyltestosterone-3-carboxymethyloxime conjugated with human serum albumin (HSA). However, the anti-serum cross-reacts with testosterone.[11] This problem may be eliminated by acetylating testosterone within the urine extracts prior to the assay. Norethandrolone, ethylestrenol (17α-ethylsteroids), and 19-nortestoster-one are detected with an antiserum directed against 19-nortestosterone-17-hemisuccinate conjugated to HSA.[14] This antiserum may give false-positive results on samples obtained from women receiving some oral contraceptives,[12] thereby emphasizing the importance of confirming im-munoassay results with GC/MS. Dugal et al.[14] used the two antisera prepared by Brooks to screen for anabolic steroids during the 1976 Montreal Olympic Games.

SOURCES OF ERROR

Three sources of error explain either a false-positive or a false-negative result. (1) Clerical error exists when the test is performed properly, but the individual or computer equipment that records and transmits the result makes an error and reports the result incorrectly. (2) Technical errors refer to situations in which the test is not performed correctly because of some human or instrumental error, and the wrong answer is obtained. The test itself may not be faulty; it was performed improperly. This reflects a lack of good quality control measures and experience. Some tests are more prone to this type of error than others; this is referred to as the reliability of the test. (3) Last, there is the error associated with collection and transportation of the samples (chain of custody). In this case, the sample arrives at the laboratory labeled with a name, but it does not belong to that person or in fact is not true urine. It is well known that a person can use many tricks to avoid submitting his or her own urine. For this reason individuals familiar with these problems believe that the sample is not worth analyzing unless a reliable person actually observes the urination.[39] The false-positive category is the most crucial of all because the person submitting the sample is considered to have used the drug in question when in fact he or she has not. Depending on how the test results are to be interpreted or used, this situation could be extremely damaging to the individual.

Any one of the errors described above can be responsible for a false-positive or a false-negative result. In addition, there is an important source of error unique to the false-negative category. A false-negative exists when the urine sample obtained from a person who has used the drug in question yields a negative test result. Obviously, the time at which the sample was collected relative to drug use must be taken into consideration. For example, if an individual gives a urine sample two hours after taking a drug and the result is negative, the test is not very useful. If the sample is collected four or five days after the last use of drug and the result is negative, it could still technically be called false-negative, but the test would not necessarily be a poor one. Thus the use of the term false-negative must always be qualified by a statement of the time elapsed since the drug was used. Likewise, it is apparent that the false-negative is related to the detection limit of the assay. An assay with a low detection limit will yield fewer false-negatives than an assay with a high detection limit.

QUALITY OF A TESTING PROGRAM

The overall quality is determined by a host of factors such as the rationale and intent of the program, prior education of the subjects, informed consent, sample collection procedures, chain of custody, laboratory procedures, sanctions, and appeals. From the perspective of the laboratory, the most important factor is avoiding false-positive results. Doping control simply cannot tolerate false positives. They are avoided by using the most definitive technique—mass spectrometry, adhering to strict laboratory protocols, using rigorous criteria for identification, using quality control samples obtained from individuals known to have received the various drugs, conservative interpretation of the data, and repeating the analysis before issuing a positive report.

Collection and clerical errors are avoided by scrupulously following a rigorous protocol. The samples are collected by specialized teams following a specific protocol that includes selecting the athletes to be tested; steps to insure that the sample is genuine urine obtained from the participant; dividing the sample into aliquot A and B; and packaging the two aliquots separately in individual zip-lock, tamper proof, transfer bags. In addition, the athlete fills out a form declaring any drugs that he or she is currently using. The laboratory conducts the analysis on the A aliquot and reports the results to the program administrators. If the result is positive, the athlete is informed and provided with an opportunity to witness the analysis of the B aliquot. At that time the B aliquot, which is still contained in the transfer bag, is inspected and the repeat analysis is observed by the athlete or a surrogate. The disposition of a positive case follows the regulations of the governing body. All organizations accept and review appeals.

ACCREDITATION BY THE INTERNATIONAL OLYMPIC COMMITTEE

The IOC/MC regulates the quality of the analyses performed by doping control laboratories by conducting accreditation examinations. The application for accreditation requests information such as a list of substances that can be identified, a list of the reference standards available to the laboratory, the minimum concentration that can be detected, the analytical equipment available, and the time required to perform a complete analysis.

The examination of the laboratory consists of analyzing 10 to 12 urine samples (unknowns) in the presence of a member of the IOC/MC.

The samples consist of human urine obtained within 24 hours of administering a conventional dose of the various drugs. Thus, the urines then contain parent drug and/or metabolites in representative amounts. The laboratory must correctly identify the unknowns within three days. An additional eight days is provided to completely document the analytical findings and submit a written report. The IOC/MC reviews the report and the observations and either issues a letter of accreditation or describes deficiencies, suggests steps to correct the deficiencies, and recommends re-examination after additional preparation.

SUMMARY

Doping agents fall into five different classes when grouped according to their major effects (Table 8–1). From the analytical perspective they may be divided into anabolic steroids and nonanabolics. The latter are usually screened for by GC, although other types of chromatography would suffice. The most definitive method of screening for anabolic steroids is GC/MS. In all cases, the finding of a drug or metabolite by a screening procedure must be confirmed by GC/MS. The finding of a substance with an RT, RRT, and mass spectrum identical to a reference standard constitutes a most definitive means of identifying a drug.

ACKNOWLEDGMENTS: This work was supported by contracts with the Los Angeles Olympic Organizing Committee and the United States Olympic Committee. I thank Caroline Hatton, Ph.D., for helpful and enlightening discussions.

REFERENCES

1. Hanley D: Drug and sex testing: Regulations for international competition. Clin Sports Med 2:13–17, 1983.
2. Oseid S: Doping and athletes— Prevention and counseling. J Allergy Clin Immunol 73:735–739, 1984.
3. Beckett AH, Cowan DA: Misuse of drugs in sport. Br J Sports Med 12:185–194, 1979.
4. Beckett AH: Drugs in sport. Br J Hosp Med 1983, pp 221–223.
5. Beckett AH: Use and abuse of drugs in sport. J Biosoc Sci Suppl 7 1981, pp 163–170.
6. Beckett AH, Tucker GT, Moffat AC: Routine detection and identification in urine of stimulants and other drugs, some of which may be used to modify performance in sport. J Pharm Pharmacol 19:273–294, 1967.
7. de Merode Prince A: Doping tests at the Olympic Games in 1976. J Sports Med 19:91–96, 1979.
8. Donike M, Kaiser CH: Moderne Methoden der Dopinganalyse. Sportarzt Sportmedizin 3:57–68, 1971.
9. Donike M: Erfahrungen mit dem Stickstoffdetektor (N-FID) bei der Dopingkontrolle. Medizinische Technik 92:153–157, 1972.
10. Donike M, Stratmann D: Temperature-programmed gas chromatographic analysis of nitrogen containing drugs: Reproducibility of retention times and sample sizes by automatic injector. Chromatographia 7:182–189, 1974.

11. Brooks RV, Firth RG, Sumner NA: Detection of anabolic steroids by radioimmunoassy. Br J Sports Med 9:89–92, 1975.
12. Brooks RV, Jeremiah G, Webb WA, Wheeler M: Detection of anabolic steroid administration to athletes. J Steroid Biochem 11:913–917, 1979.
13. Bertrand M, Masse R, Dugal R: GC-MS approach for the detection and characterization of anabolic steroids and their metabolites in biological fluids at major international sporting events. Farmaceutische Tijdschrift Belgie 3:85–101, 1978.
14. Dugal R, Dupuis C, Bertrand MJ: Radioimmunoassay of anabolic steroids: An evaluation of three antisera for the detection of anabolic steroids in biological fluids. Br J Sports Med 11:162–169, 1977.
15. Personal communication: Prince A. de Merode, Chairman, IOC Medical Commission, May, 1985.
16. Faraj BA, Israli ZH, Perel JM, et al: Metabolism and disposition of methylphenidate-14C: Studies in man and animals. J Pharmacol Exp Ther 191:535–547, 1974.
17. Bastos ML, Jukofsky D, Mule SJ: Routine identification of cocaine metabolites in human urine. J Chromatogr 89:335–342, 1974.
18. Durbeck MW, Buker I, Scheulen B, et al: Gas chromatographic and capillary column gas chromatographic-mass spectrometric determination of synthetic anabolic steroids. I. Methanedinone and its metabolites. J Chromatogr 167:117–124, 1978.
19. Bjorkhem I, Lantto O, Lof A: Detection and quantitation of methandienone (Dianabol) in urine by isotope dilution-mass fragmentography. J Steroid Biochem 13:169–175, 1980.
20. Bjorkhem I, Ek H: Detection and quantitation of 19-norandrosterone in urine by isotope dilution-mass spectrometry. J Steroid Biochem 17:447–451, 1982.
21. Bjorkhem I, Ek H: Detection and quantitation of 3-hydroxy-1-methylen-5-androstan-17-one. The major urinary metabolite of methenolone (Primobolan) by isotope dilution-mass spectrometry. J Steroid Biochem 18:481–487, 1983.
22. Gottheil E, Caddy GR, Austin DL: Fallibility of urine drug screens in monitoring methadone programs. JAMA 236:1035–1038, 1976.
23. Hansen HJ, Caudill SP, Boone DJ: Crisis in drug testing. JAMA 253:2382–2387, 1985.
24. Willard HH, Merritt LL, Dean JA, Settle FA: Chromatography—General principles. In Instrumental Methods of Analysis. New York, Van Nostrand Reinhold, 1981.
25. Sherma J, Fried B: Thin-layer and paper chromatography. Anal Chem 56:48R–63R, 1984.
26. Majors RE, Barth HG, Lochmuller CH: Column liquid chromatography. Anal Chem 56:300R–349R, 1984.
27. Karasek FW, Onuska FI, Yang FJ, Clement RE: Gas chromatography. Anal Chem 56:174R–199R, 1984.
28. Marozzi E, Gambaro V, Saligari E, Mariani R, Lodi F: Use of the retention index in gas chromatographic studies of drugs. J Anal Toxicol 6:185–192, 1982.
29. Burlingame AL, Whitney JO, Russell DH: Mass spectrometry. Anal Chem 56:417R–447R, 1984.
30. Gaskell SJ: Analysis of steroids by mass spectrometry. Methods Biochem Anal 29:385–434, 1983.
31. Bjorkhem I: Selective ion monitoring in clinical chemistry. CRC Crit Rev Clin Lab Sci 11:53–105, 1979.
32. Donike M, Zimmermann J, Barwald KR, Schanzer W, Christ V, Klostermann Opfermann G: Routinebestimmung von Anabolika im Harn. Dtsch Z Sportmedizin 35:14–24, 1984.
33. Houghton E, Teale P: Capillary column gas chromatographic mass spectrometric analysis of anabolic steroid residues using splitless injections made at elevated temperatures. Biomed Mass Spectrom 8:358–361, 1981.
34. Donike M: Trifluoroacetyl-0-trimethylsilyl-phenolalkylamines. Preparation and gas chromatographic estimation. J Chromatogr 103:91–112, 1975.
35. Skelley DS, Brown LP, Besch PK: Radioimmunoassay. Clin Chem 19:146–186, 1973.
36. Zettner A: Principles of competitive binding assays (saturation analyses). I. Equilibrium techniques. Clin Chem 19:699–705, 1973.

37. Jondorf RW: 19-Nortestosterone, a model for the use of anabolic steroid conjugates in raising antibodies for radioimmunoassay. Xenobiotica 7:671–681, 1977.

38. Hampl R, Starka L: Practical aspects of screening of anabolic steroids in doping control with particular accent to nortestosterone radioimmunoassay using mixed antisera. J Steroid Biochem 11:933–939, 1979.

39. Goldstein A, Brown BW: Urine testing schedules in methadone maintenance treatment of heroin addiction. JAMA 214:311–315, 1970.

9

PSYCHOLOGICAL AIDS
TO PERFORMANCE

ROD K. DISHMAN, PH.D.

Thoughts (cognition), emotion (affect), and sensations (perception) influence human performance in measurable and systematic ways.[1, 2] This has spurred the search for psychological and behavioral interventions that can be applied in competitive sport settings. The objective is to predictably enhance athletic achievement in a manner that complements existing methods from instructional (coaching and conditioning), nutritional, and medical services. In this chapter I describe the cornerstone principles, technologies, and factual base that undergird present-day use of psychology as an athletic aid.

Psychological interventions in sport are commonly *acute;* the goal is to temporarily augment motivation or skill so that a performance exceeds an expected standard established by prior performances. When medical, physiological, or biomechanical factors appear unchanged, an atypical performance can usually be attributed to a psychological origin. Psychological aids can also be *chronic,* where the focus is on long-term outcomes and preparation, not just readiness before or during a contest. In either the acute or chronic case, it is useful to consider circumstances in which nonpsychological components of performance (e.g., health, fitness, or technique) can be affected by psychological or behavioral events. This view helps define objective mechanisms through which psychology can impact on sport outcomes, and it helps trace variability in physical and biomedical factors that is otherwise unexplained.

Psychological interventions can be designed not only to augment performance above an expected level (by enhancing or adding skills) but to elevate an artificially suppressed performance back to an expected level (by diminishing temporary barriers). Thus, psychological techniques can be both developmental (educational) and therapeutic, and application of the intervention can originate from a professional (in the form of a service) or from the athlete (in the form of self-regulation). The targets can be enhanced skills and capacities or their normal expression. Although the ergogenic success of interventions is gauged by objectively measured outcomes, the influence of psychological or behavioral events in sport often hinges on subjective (self-defined) goals and appraisals; in this way psychology is unique among performance-enhancing phenomena.

Key psychological factors include those that economize the direction and optimize the magnitude of motivation.[2] Attainable and effective career, seasonal, and contest goals must be established for both conditioning and peak performance, while incentives and reinforcement must be present so that optimal effort is sustained but not exceeded in a way that promotes injury or overtraining. Thoughts, feelings, and behaviors that hinder performance or health must be diminished. In these ways an athlete is able to use existing or developing talent effectively. Equally important are psychological aids that directly influence skills and capacities in ways beyond those predicted by general principles of physiology or technique. Selective processing of sensory information from the sport environment, decision-making for strategic and well-timed movements, and precise execution of motor plans with suitable direction, force, power, and endurance are all sensitive to transient and chronic central nervous system functions that can be assessed by cognitive, affective, and perceptual measures.[3, 4] Thus they are, in part, psychological skills. While they are affected by physiology and clearly reflect stable or enduring traits attributable to genotype, maturation, and experience, psychological skills are believed to also be sensitive to changes induced by systematic behavioral instruction and acute psychological intervention.

This is convincingly seen when portions of performance outcomes usually attributed to other ergogenic techniques are equally well explained by psychology.[2] For example, the impact of prior activity (e.g., warm-up) on both metabolic (ventilation, heart rate, cardiac output, oxygen consumption) and motoric (reaction time, force, movement precision) components of performance is well-established. Yet, study has shown this effect can be mediated by an individual's beliefs or attitudes toward warm-up. In one early investigation[5] employing bicycle ergometry, the use of hypnotic amnesia as a control for subjects' conscious awareness of a warm-up period indicated that the warm-up per se had no effect on subsequent performance.

TARGETS FOR PSYCHOLOGICAL INTERVENTIONS

Although many other types of sport behaviors are probably important to performance outcomes and are sensitive to psychological events, available evidence can be organized around metabolic parameters, strength and endurance, skilled movements, and behaviors that occur outside the competitive setting but support competitive success.

METABOLIC PARAMETERS

A facilitative influence of beliefs on warm-up effects is consistent with other controlled research using hypnotic or waking suggestions of emotions, work, and relaxation under actual resting or exercise conditions. During the waking, resting state, merely contracting facial muscles to mimic emotion prototypes for anger or fear has led to an 8-bpm increase in heart rate.[6] Imagined emotional states of anger and fear during rest have also increased heart rate (10 bpm) and systolic blood pressure (6 to 7 mm Hg).[7] Years ago, it was reported that pre-event anticipatory increases in heart rate accounted for 59 per cent of the total heart-rate adjustment during footracing among young girls.[8] In a related laboratory study, hypnotically imagined exercise induced an elevation in heart rate that was 57 per cent of that measured (42 bpm above rest) during an actual 10-minute treadmill bout at 3 mph and 5 per cent grade.[9] Morgan has reported in a recent review[4] that hypnotic suggestions of light and heavy work made to resting subjects have increased oxygen consumption by 92 to 409 ml $\cdot$ min^{-1}, ventilatory minute volume by 4.0 to 19.3 l $\cdot$ min^{-1}, heart rate by 10 to 40 bpm, and cardiac output by 4.7 l $\cdot$ min^{-1}. Studies of hypnotically hallucinated exercise during rest have also demonstrated elevations in blood lipids and several of the stress hormones that help regulate metabolic adjustments during exercise.

Similar results can occur during exercise. Convincing data by Morgan and his colleagues[10, 11] have shown that during 5 minutes of stationary bicycling at a constant power of 100 watts, hypnotic suggestions of heavy exercise can result in increased perceptions of exertion, a 15 bpm increase in heart rate, and a 15-liter increase in ventilatory minute volume when contrasted with waking control responses at the same intensity. Similarly, at a constant power of 100 watts, when hypnotic suggestions of 5 minutes of "uphill" exercise followed 10 minutes of suggested "level" exercise, a significant elevation in perceived exertion occurred. This was accompanied by an increase in minute ventilation of 10 liters above control conditions. In the waking state, imagined emotions of anger and fear have augmented the typical increases in heart rate (by 12 to 19 bpm) and systolic blood pressure (by 12 to 13 mm Hg) that accompany light bench stepping (40 cm for 1 min).[7] Conversely, studies inducing standardized relaxation procedures during exercise have reported reductions in oxygen consumption of 4 per cent (0.763 to 0.730 l $\cdot$ min^{-1})[12] and 9 per cent (0.800 to 0.720 l $\cdot$ min^{-1})[13] during continuous (8- and 10-minute) stationary bicycling (heart rates were constant at 95 and 115 bpm) in nonathletes and 12 per cent (36.7 to 32.1 ml $\cdot$ kg^{-1} $\cdot$ min^{-1})[14] during continuous (20-minute) treadmill running (50 per cent $\dot{V}O_2$ max) in college cross-country athletes.

The magnitude of these reductions is not, however, consistent with studies employing more prolonged or intense exercise, and it is doubtful that a psychological state can alone increase the acute metabolic efficiency of an experienced runner to an extent that approximates the total variability in efficiency seen among both competitive (12 per cent) and recreational (17 per cent) runners.[15] The practical performance or medical significance of these types of metabolic changes is likely restricted to ultra-endurance events, hostile environments (e.g., temperature and humidity extremes), and patients with cardiopulmonary or metabolic disorders. In each case, emotional stress could compound, or psychological skills might ease, existing strain to a meaningful extent. At any rate, the observation that *imagined* work can produce a physiological arousal similar in form and approaching the magnitude of actual prior exercise of light or moderate intensities is consistent with a potentiating effect for thoughts, emotions, and perceptions on performance.

MUSCULAR STRENGTH AND ENDURANCE

Early study[16] using hypnotic suggestions of strength or weakness has shown even greater increases (26 per cent) and decreases (31 per cent) in the expression of force when contrasted with pharmacological ergogens, where increases ranged from 6 to 14 per cent for alcohol, amphetamine, and epinephrine. However, hypnotic suggestions of strength or muscular endurance typically show best results for nonathletes, because athletes usually are already relatively close to top performance owing to training and high motivation. For these reasons, measures of strength and endurance are highly stable in athletes and conditioned individuals. On the other hand, even among competitive weight lifters, the use of mental preparation strategies in the waking state has increased the expression of force by 5 to 10 per cent above baseline "maxima,"[17] and controlled cases of phenomenal endurance breakthroughs by well-conditioned athletes after post-hypnotic suggestions are convincingly documented. In one case,[18] hypnotic suggestions of decreased fatigue enabled a professional football player to increase his endurance at a 47-lb bench press from a previous best of 130 repetitions to 233. On a subsequent day in the waking state he was stopped by the investigators at 350 repetitions!

Among young untrained adults, motivating conditions or contrived performance expectations can typically lead to a 5 to 15 per cent transient increase in muscular force and endurance.[2, 17] A simple attentional distraction and relaxation technique known as dissociation has increased self-limited treadmill endurance by 20 per cent among healthy young males even in the absence of measurable metabolic or biochemical changes.[19] And in field tests,[20] which are based on performance, and symptom-limited treadmill tests[21] where expired gases are measured, 12 to 18 per cent of aerobic power can be explained by psychological traits related to motivation. Such results argue strongly for a psychology of human performance that might be systematically altered.

MOTOR SKILLS

The role of psychological interventions in sport extends beyond the expression of functional capacities, however. Metabolic parameters, force, and endurance permit objective and highly reliable measurements and have profound impacts on sport performance. But success in many sports depends equally or more on complex skills related to processing sensory information from the sport environment, decision making, and precise movement. In fact, evidence suggests performance skills of these types originate more in cortical functions of the central nervous system than do performance components of force, work, and power.[3] Anxiety and depressed moods can narrow or distract concentration and increase muscle tension so that environmental cues are missed, strategies are forgotten, and precise movement patterns are broken. The accompanying avoidance behaviors and dampened confidence can block the expression of existing skills and retard the development of new ones. Conversely, when thoughts of poor ability or likely failure are replaced by expected success and are augmented by energizing moods (pride or competence are at stake), performance can be optimized. In many instances, however, high-level performance is associated with the absence of conscious decision making; at times, the goal in sports is to remove psychology, not change it.

Although clearly important for performance, complex skills are difficult to measure objectively. Performance ratings by judges are unreliable, outcome statistics obscure underlying skills, while component or segmental analyses of movement (kinetics and kinematics) describe differences in technique but seldom predict success among high-level performers. Despite these difficulties, the performance potential for psychological interventions is perhaps greatest in complex skills, where small variations in precision or consistency are keys to successful outcomes.

SUPPORT BEHAVIORS

Behaviors outside the competitive setting that enable skills and fitness to develop or to be maintained in healthy and performance-enhancing ways are also targets for psychological intervention. Examples in this category include athletic conditioning, eating behaviors and substance use, interpersonal relations (with family, coaches, peers, and management personnel), and academic study habits (for school and college athletes). Problems and interventions in these behaviors have only recently been studied,[22-24] so very little about them is known.[1]

PSYCHOLOGICAL INTERVENTIONS

An ultimate target of all psychological interventions is behavior, although approaches differ fundamentally in their views of the origins of behavior. This leads to procedures that vary widely in methods and techniques, and the debate over which are most effective remains active. The preferences of a given psychologist or psychiatrist are likely to reflect training as much as a decision made on scientific evidence of efficacy or the specific problem or athlete that is encountered.

BEHAVIORISM

Behaviorism regards behavior as a function of observable response to objective events in the environment. The emphasis is on reproducible changes in behavior or neuroendocrine symptoms that result from associations between an external stimulus and an action. Responses can be classically conditioned (Pavlovian) to a single experience (e.g., some phobic and somatic disturbances) or operantly conditioned (to achieve a goal) through repeated pairing with a consequent event (a reinforcer) or an extraneous event (a secondary reinforcer) that increases (reinforcement) or decreases (punishment) the likelihood of the response in the future. This forms the basis of most behavior modification approaches.[25]

Desired behaviors can often be altered quickly by continuous reinforcement or modified in a more long-lasting way by an intermittent schedule. Common behavioristic procedures include the following: (1) *Shaping:* Existing behaviors similar to the desired behavior or sub-parts of a desired behavior that is complex are progressively reinforced; or a behavior exhibited in many undesired settings is reinforced in one or only a few desired settings. (2) *Generalizing:* A behavior exhibited in a single setting is gradually reinforced when it is shown elsewhere; or additional desired behaviors related to an existing one are reinforced in the initial setting. (3) *Fading:* Reinforcement or punishment by a professional of a desired behavior is gradually made less frequent or less intense so that self-reinforcement or punishment by the client/athlete is increased. These are typically implemented by techniques such as *reinforcement* or *punishment control* (e.g., social evaluation, feedback, prize lotteries, contingency contracts or tokens, awards, written agreements, withholding rewards, or pain) or *stimulus control* (whereby naturally occurring secondary reinforcers are structured to cue or prompt the desired behavior). Examples of widely used therapeutic techniques[25, 27] include the following: (1) *Systematic desensitization*[26] counterconditions avoidance behaviors and emotions by a graduated pairing of aversive situations or images with responses, such as progressive relaxation or task mastery, that are incompatible with the aversive state. (2) *Flooding* attempts to force an adaptive response or extinguish one that is maladaptive by preventing avoidance from real or imagined aversive situations.

Behavioristic procedures are known to effectively treat numerous behavioral and somatic disorders that are of clinical significance. They appear compatible with the instructional and motivational methods used intuitively by many successful athletic coaches. However, despite several books that describe sport application,[28–30] there are relatively few empirical studies to demonstrate the impact of behavioral methods on sports performance.[31] There are reports of increases in athletes' workout behaviors and training volume in swimming, basketball, weightlifting, and volleyball; enhanced execution of existing offensive skills in baseball and American football; and altered verbal behaviors (such as goal-focused encouragement) by both coaches and team members. Behavioristic techniques have also been used recently as coaching adjuncts in the acquisition of beginning and intermediate skill levels for golf, football, gymnastics, soccer, tennis, and track sprinting.[32-34]

Although these studies are encouraging, they have largely been case studies dealing with support behaviors or with technique at relatively low levels of skill or experience. In many instances their effectiveness was compared with what appeared to be poor coaching instruction that had little chance of being effective. Reports of therapeutic applications with athletes experiencing clinical problems are not widespread. Even though the use of time-series designs in some studies enhances their internal validity (e.g., the outcomes appear directly linked to the intervention), alternative explanations such as therapist effects (e.g., not what is done, but how or by whom) and Hawthorne effects (any treatment is better than none) typically have not been discounted. Also, inferential statistics have seldom been used to decide the significance of the changes observed. Thus, the ability to reproduce and generalize reported outcomes for other athletes or settings is unclear. This makes it difficult to estimate their real performance impact.

A key to the effectiveness of behavioristic intervention lies in identifying critical behaviors. This can be relatively straightforward for simple support behaviors such as physical conditioning or study habits, and a qualified therapist is trained to do this for clinical disorders. On the other hand, isolating sub-components for technique enhancement at high skill-levels requires specialized knowledge and experience in the sport, and indeed, this often exceeds the state-of-knowledge in sports science. Finding effective reinforcers for different athletes can also be a problem, and the existence of individual differences in reinforcement potency is a serious limitation for standardized applications of behaviorism to sport settings.

BIOFEEDBACK

Biofeedback involves a technological interface (e.g., visual or auditory analogues) between external senses, the conscious (e.g., voluntary) nervous system, and the autonomic nervous system.[27] In this way, information about biological states that would otherwise be undetected is made available to a patient's/client's awareness. In principle, this can allow an individual to acquire a degree of self-control over typically autonomic functions (e.g., heart rate, blood pressure, electrical potentials in brain and striate muscle). Biofeedback has been applied as a therapy, mostly in behavioral medicine, for about 15 years. Its clinical use stemmed largely from the prevalence of stress-related somatic disorders in the population and from converging interests by behaviorism, learning psychology, and psychophysiology in whether autonomic nervous system responses could be shaped by operant procedures rather than conditioned exclusively by classical methods (Pavlovian procedures).[35] Although early study argued that visceral responses could be operantly controlled apart from intrinsic fusimotor feedback or mechanical influence by striate muscle, this finding has not been consistently replicated and is currently debated. Early findings showing that biofeedback-induced reductions in heart rate during a constant exercise intensity depended on autonomic perception by the subjects were recently not reproduced by the same investigators under the same laboratory conditions.[36]

Biofeedback-assisted learning in sport has primarily involved control of neuromuscular tension.[37] Biofeedback of frontalis electromyograms has been associated with decreased tension and improved gross balance (stabilometer) and fine motor precision (pursuit rotor) for undergraduates when compared to control and placebo conditions. But no changes in stabilometer performance was reported when tension was reduced among a group of trait anxious boys. In more complex skills, no performance effects were observed for novice archers (target accuracy) or novice underwater divers (underwater assembly), despite reduced tension in the frontalis. Similarly, for competitive athletes, biofeedback assisted (EMG) frontalis relaxation had no effects on subjective anxiety or competitive gymnastic scores for age-level females (when combined with progressive relaxation) or college males (when combined with systematic desensitization), although frontalis tension was reduced for the males. Coaches' ratings of performance for college football players (raters were not blinded) and college basketball players (raters were blinded) were improved when frontalis tension was reduced by frontalis EMG feedback (combined with cognitive restructuring and heart rate feedback). Compared with a placebo, auditory feedback of heart rate and respiration increased the reliability of their synchronous patterning with target accuracy among national caliber rifle shooters.

As for many clinical procedures, the prevalence of biofeedback seems to have outstripped established principles to ensure its effective application. Guides for learning through biofeedback (e.g., the preferred modality or the time course required for retention) remain inadequately documented by empirical data. Information about sports applications is limited in several other ways. Most studies have used biofeedback to reduce neuromuscular symptoms of stress without first determining if a particular level of muscular tension is optimal for performance in the sport studied and without considering performance enhancing patterns of response for individual athletes. Personality factors that influence tension levels, performance, or the ability to learn have essentially been ignored. The frontalis muscle has been used in most studies, apparently because it is responsive to feedback, but its patterning is known to be poorly correlated with that of skeletal muscle and subjective anxiety. Although frontalis EMG feedback can acutely affect other systems (e.g., HR, BP), it is doubtful these changes persist. This makes it difficult to explain why tension reduction in the frontalis would enhance performance in the sports studied.

The effectiveness of biofeedback appears to depend on matching the symptom of interest with its control pathway in the CNS. Yet with few exceptions, sports studies of biofeedback have not first demonstrated which somatic factors, or their patterning, were related to performance levels of the subjects studied or they have not studied athletes with a history of clinical symptoms. Systems other than muscle tension and techniques besides EMG have received little attention, and the use of biofeedback to directly enhance performance (e.g., shape movement precision or timing, augment neuromuscular conditioning or rehabilitation) has not been widely reported. Importantly, studies have not documented that learning to control autonomic systems under resting or precompetitive conditions will extend to voluntary control during the acute demands of ongoing competition.

COGNITIVE-BEHAVIORAL PROCEDURES

Behaviorism and somatic procedures (e.g., biofeedback, progressive relaxation,[38] and anxiolytic drugs[39]) minimize the role of thoughts, emotions, and perceptions in determining behavior. The emphasis is on objective situations and overt responses. While sociology and pharmacology have revealed that we share many common behaviors and bodily responses, it is equally clear that many people do not respond in identical ways to the same situations. Not only can humans learn without being reinforced (e.g., by observation), but evidence confirms we are motivated for future efforts by knowledge of behavior outcomes and future expectations. It can be argued that past stimulus-response-reinforcement patterns account for individual variations in current situational responses. However, study confirms that perceptions, emotions, and thoughts account for significant portions of present-day variations in the reinforcement value of objective events. And these subjective patterns are often more readily identified than are critical histories. Most people have characteristic ways in which they experience thoughts and emotions in many situations. Thus, methods designed to change them should allow for more broadreaching outcomes than behavioristic procedures that are bound to a single or narrow range of stimulus-response associations.

This has led some psychologists to modify the learning principles and techniques developed by behaviorism for overt behaviors so they can be used with covert behaviors such as anxiety or depression, self-confidence, and motivation.[40] The use of aversive images in systematic desensitization[26] is an early example of this approach. Yet this is based on counterconditioning principles and is designed for single behaviors. The underlying assumption of more recently developed cognitive-behavioral procedures is that a wide range of dysfunctional or maladaptive behaviors stem from the development of irrational and unproductive thoughts and beliefs or incompletely formed cognitions. It is believed that by applying learning principles, or sometimes by providing the client with insight, faulty thoughts can be restructured and augmented or replaced by beliefs and cognitive skills that are behaviorally more effective.

These approaches typically share common stages even though their characteristic features vary. There is an initial stage during which the professional *probes* the thoughts and belief systems of the client/patient and determines the behavioral habits that result. This is followed by an *educational stage* that fosters in the individual expectancies of change and evaluates possible plans that can promote change. Next comes a stage when the actual treatment *plan is designed*. Finally, an attempt is made to *implement and maintain* the plan in daily life. Relapse[41] is common, however, so there is frequently a return to earlier stages among those who have difficulty changing but retain the desire to change.

Several procedures rely nearly exclusively on eliminating or restructuring thought. It is assumed that desired changes in behavior or emotion will follow but neither are direct targets of the interventions. This is a radically different view from behaviorism or biofeedback where the emphasis excludes conscious mediators of behavioral or somatic responses.

Rational emotive therapy (RET)[42] is a forerunner of modern day cognitive psychotherapy, which attempts to substitute rational thoughts for the illogical or exaggerated beliefs people hold about life events and interpersonal relations. At the core of irrational thinking are the misattribution of cause to the wrong source and the absolute expectations of others or oneself that unavoidably create self-fulfilling prophecies of disappointments, misplaced blame, and negative emotion. The founder of RET, Albert Ellis, refers to many faulty assumptions as "musts" or "have to's." Examples are: (A) I must be totally competent in every way in order to be a worthwhile person. (B) I have to be loved or approved of by everyone. (C) When things don't go my way, it is a catastrophe. (D) Bad feelings are out of my control, and when something is threatening I must keep thinking it might happen. The key to RET is insight that often it is not the objective event but the set of beliefs one holds about the source of the event and its consequences that leads to aversive emotions and avoidance behavior. If these beliefs can be changed, so too will negative responses.

Other popular cognitive therapies[43] are based on restructuring maladaptive beliefs formed by biased or incomplete attention to all the feedback from a behavior (e.g., a little criticism is given more weight than a lot of praise) or when a conclusion is reached in the absence of real events (neurotic speculation).

Examples of cognitive restructuring are *thought stopping*[44] (obsessive or neurotic patterns of recurrent thoughts are interrupted by counterconditioning the onset of a negative self-dialogue with a blocking cue such as an innocuous word) and *positive self-talk* (a neurotic or self-defeating internal dialogue is replaced by one that is rational or that prompts a desired action). In these ways, thoughts that trigger maladaptive behaviors or that prevent adaptive ones can be eliminated or substituted by positive thoughts. Cognitive therapies are most commonly employed in treating unipolar, neurotic depression and its associated cognitive anxiety when somatic therapies are not indicated.

Because the proportion of competitive athletes who experience depressive episodes approximates general population rates, cognitive psychotherapy is a viable therapeutic alternative in sport. However, reports of psychotherapy with athletes are not widespread.[45] There are also few studies that evaluate the performance impact of thought stopping, internal dialogues, or cognitive restructuring in mentally healthy athletes.[37] Collectively, findings on thought stopping or restructuring in sport indicate that the procedures were effective in changing the covert behaviors targeted, but performance was not affected. These studies did not, however, control for skill levels (if there is no documented performance decrement, room for improvement may be small) or did not test athletes experiencing maladaptive ruminations. Case study of performance slumps have, however, shown elevated performance.[46] Internal dialogue seems to exert a more robust impact on performance than does thought restructuring, but again there are few studies with athletes in sports settings. And it is unclear whether the effects seen are instructional (e.g., strategy or technique), confidence building, or motivating in nature. In most instances, cognitive methods in sport have been imbedded in broader intervention packages that include behavioral or somatic components. This practice may augment clinical outcomes, but it precludes an independent evaluation of impact for cognitive changes. Also, cognitive therapies fail to consider that for emotionally stable and confident personalities, self-critical thoughts can be both instructive and motivating.

Hypnosis[27] can be viewed as a cognitive technique that can be useful in gaining personal insights less accessible in the waking state. Although hypnosis is generally regarded as an altered state of consciousness, its effectiveness for influencing behaviors or skills depends on the suggestions used. This effect does not appear to exceed that of the waking state when suggestible individuals have their performance expectancies changed or when motivating incentives are present. There is no convincing evidence that a hypnotized person will demonstrate skills or behaviors that do not already exist in latent form during waking circumstances. The usefulness of hypnosis as a standardized aid in sport is limited because people vary widely in responsiveness and the time needed to learn how to enter a deep trance. No more than 20 per cent are believed capable of easily entering a somnamnic state. An equal number are chronically resistive. For some personalities there are psychological risks that accompany hypnosis (e.g., insights may confront deep conflicts, normal values might be violated, the client may become dependent on the therapist), and for this reason it should be used only under the supervision of a qualified professional (ideally this might be one certified by the American Board of Psychological Hypnosis).

The experimental use of hypnotic suggestion to alter strength, endurance, and metabolic parameters was discussed earlier in this chapter and elsewhere.[2, 4] Collectively, findings indicate that hypnosis per se has little reliable impact on performance, but hypnotic suggestions designed to either enhance or impede performance are quite effective. However, suggestions in the hypnotic state appear no more effective than those made to subjects in the motivated, waking state. Laboratory studies of hypnosis and skilled performance[47] have been limited to contrived tasks such as ball bouncing, mirror tracing, scores on reaction time, and stylus maze apparatus. As found for functional capacities, fine motor skills can be positively or negatively influenced by hypnosis, but the effects are mediated by the suggestions used. Those that alter arousal or alertness in a manner compatible with the skill requirements for concentration and movement precision are likely to be most effective for enhancing performance.

Although less standardized or generalized, the greatest potential for hypnosis in sports may be as a clinical adjunct for treating personal or sports-related problems on an individual athlete basis. While anecdotal reports of performance breakthroughs are widespread and are probably exaggerated or misinterpreted in many instances, there are numerous case studies that report successful remediation of performance slumps following hypnotic sessions.[47] These range from self-analysis of a technique problem in baseball hitting, resolution of aggression conflicts in contact sports, control of performance anxiety, removal of neurotic barriers to the rehabilitation of injury, and the use of hypnosis to aid in the recall and conditioning of optimal performance arousal.

SELF-REGULATION AND COPING SKILLS

During the past decade increasing emphasis has been placed on self-regulation of thoughts, emotions, and behavior by the patient/client. This is partly because a large portion of modern-day disorders apparently stem from the daily hassles and free-floating stress of living in an era where more and more goals are pursued in less and less time. The relatively radical clinical methods founded in behaviorism or early psychotherapy for abnormal psychology were not designed to cope with more transient and less severe neurotic episodes that, though not disabling, diminish a productive and enjoyable life. Modern day cognitive-behavioral procedures[27] not only identify problem thoughts or situations, but they emphasize the acquisition of coping skills that the person can apply when situations require them. The construction of an active plan for behavior (an adaptive alternative) separates these techniques from behavioristic, somatic, or cognitive approaches that focus primarily on eliminating maladaptive responses.

This instructional focus makes cognitive-behavioral procedures attractive for sports applications. The majority of performance problems in sports are not pathological in origin; thus applications often do not require clinical training. And self-regulation permits the athlete to develop skills for responding to the dynamic demands of ongoing competition; the goal is skill development more than acute therapy.

In *stress inoculation*,[48] coping skills (progressive muscle relaxation and adaptive self-statements) are rehearsed amid conditions of low anxiety or aversion that are manageable for the client. It is assumed this mastery will then extend to real-life environments where stress has been excessive. Thus the individual is inoculated in a way that is analogous to antigen-antibody reactions. The direction of the effect is somewhat akin to that of systematic desensitization, although the gradation from low- to high-anxiety situations is largely up to the client.

In *cognitive-affective stress management*,[49] however, high levels of emotion are induced so that the coping response is rehearsed under imagined conditions that simulate or exceed real world stress. This approach more approximates flooding procedures; the goal is to extinguish the avoidance response, although this is attempted consciously. The subject is taught to block the imagined emotional peak through self-instruction. In early stages this is accomplished by somatic means using progressive muscle relaxation. Later, rational self-statements are used. Finally, both the somatic and cognitive relaxation techniques are synchronized with the breathing cycle in a way similar to Bensonian meditation.[50]

The use of stress inoculation and cognitive-affective stress management with athletes has not been widely reported.[51] Yet each should be as effective in dealing with stress-related disorders experienced by athletes as they would for nonathletes when problems are of a clinical nature. The degree to which personalities or circumstances peculiar to sports might compromise their effectiveness is not known. However, it is believed that in subclinical instances, sports outcomes might still be enhanced if the self-instruction components contained self-statements to cue and monitor technique, strategy, and concentration.

As defined by Bandura,[52] *self-efficacy* is the confidence one has in executing a specific behavior when the outcome is known. This feature distinguishes self-efficacy from other confidence factors that depend on uncertainties about outcome or are designed to account for behavior in many settings. Self-efficacy is also independent of incentives for the behavior. This distinguishes it from perceived competence in which self-esteem both shapes confidence and motivates behavior. According to Bandura, self-efficacy is a cognitive factor that determines the direction, effort, and persistence of behavior and is formed by actual past performance accomplishments, observation of performance by others, verbal persuasion, and sensations of emotional arousal that signal ability rather than anxiety. The strength and generalizability of self-efficacy are dependent on behavioral, observational, and cognitive learning principles, yet behavior is viewed as ultimately cognitive in origin.

This feature has been attractive for sports psychologists, but it has been widely criticized by clinical psychologists whose methods are based more in behavioristic principles.[53] Critics argue that self-efficacy does not determine anxiety and performance responses; rather, anxiety reduction leads to enhanced performance and thus to higher self-efficacy.

Several sport and exercise experiments have shown that circumstances contrived to increase self-efficacy (e.g., client-aided or observed modeling, manipulated self-expectancy) can lead to transient increases in the expression of muscular strength, endurance, and performance in high-avoidance skills such as springboard diving and gymnastic stunts.[17, 37] Although these studies confirm that self-efficacy is associated with performance in high-risk skills (particularly with the novice), they also indicate that performance is predicted by past successes or failures and by physiological indices of anxiety. In fact, self-efficacy in sports appears to depend as much on past performance as future performance depends on self-efficacy.[54, 55] These findings are important for choosing preferred sports interventions, because they support behavioristic views of anxiety as much as cognitive-based models of self-confidence.

PSYCHOLOGICAL INTERVENTIONS DESIGNED FOR SPORTS

Cognitive-behavioral interventions have generally not demonstrated behavioral outcomes that are as pronounced as behavioristic procedures. This might be expected because by definition the primary targets are thoughts and emotions. Although this issue is highly relevant for evaluating their potential for ergogenic purposes, it is still important to consider instances when an athlete's well-being is enhanced even though behavior or performance might remain unchanged.

Other approaches have adapted cognitive-behavioral techniques like the aforementioned to be used specifically as performance aids among apparently healthy athletes. In these applications, the intervention targets are principally sport skills (e.g., concentration, tension control) instead of cognitive or affective symptoms of stress emotions.

ATTENTION CONTROL TRAINING

Attention control training (ACT) by Nideffer[56] integrates the learning of selective attention to crucial technique and setting cues with anxiety and tension control. The principal goal is to prevent shifts in attention that do not satisfy performance demands of a particular sport. The underlying theoretical model conceptualizes attention along independent continua of narrow-to-broad width and internal-to-external focus. The assumption is that the attentional style an athlete typically employs may be counterproductive to the attentional demands of the sport. Experimental laboratory research supports the importance of attentional focus, and cross-sectional studies confirm that both general and sport-specific attentional styles can distinguish athletes according to their sport and success levels.[37] Although ACT is a popular application, reports on its effectiveness for altering attentional styles and performance have not been widespread.

VISUO-MOTOR BEHAVIOR REHEARSAL

Visuo-motor behavior rehearsal (VMBR) is a technique developed by Suinn[57] that is adapted from the imagery and relaxation instructions underlying Wolpe's systematic desensitization.[26] Its cognitive component is designed to enhance performance by using imagined technique rehearsal or goals to cue the execution of performance. This is accompanied by self-regulated anxiety management to increase or diminish emotional arousal according to the performance needs of a given athlete or sport skill.

VMBR has been the most widely tested cognitive-behavioral procedure applied in sport settings.[37, 40] Controlled and uncontrolled case studies have shown improved match play in golf and game performance by a placekicker in American football, while a study of competitive free throw percentage among college male basketball players showed those assigned to VMBR improved, whereas those assigned to relaxation, imagery, or control groups did not. A controlled study of VMBR with amateur tennis players reported no performance effects, even though tension levels were reduced (EMG). Similarly, a pre-post comparison of competitive performance among groups of college golfers and runners after VMBR showed no effects.

In each of these studies it was assumed that performance would be aided by decreased anxiety, increased confidence, and more focused attention. Yet these factors were not assessed. In group settings it seems unlikely that general standardized instructions and procedures for VMBR will be equally effective for all athletes, because performance needs and the ability to learn and employ VMBR will surely vary among individuals. A recent well-controlled study of beginning karate students[58] has shown that individualized VMBR was more effective in enhancing performance than were placebo or nonindividualized conditions, but a programmed learning package developed by Suinn was also effective.

The necessary time for an effective VMBR intervention remains unclear, however. Several studies have not specified the time spent, while in others it has varied from three 50-minute sessions to fifteen 10- to 20-minute sessions every day for six weeks. Furthermore, less than half the published studies using VMBR as the intervention have reported employing placebo groups as a control for generalized expectancies of benefits by the subjects. Thus it is often not possible to conclude that VMBR effects simply exceeded no intervention. Most studies have not included manipulation checks to estimate the extent to which the imagery and relaxation skills of VMBR are actually invoked during practice sessions, are learned, or are transferred to competitive settings.

Other studies[37] have embedded VMBR within comprehensive cognitive-behavior modification packages (e.g., stress inoculation and thought stopping) for the needs of individual athletes in college basketball and amateur tennis or for group application (with cognitive restructuring) among college gymnasts, archers, wrestlers, badminton players, and cross-country skiers. Performance results in these studies are mixed, but the impact of VMBR cannot be evaluated because it was confounded with other interventions.

Collectively, studies showing performance increases following VMBR do not specify the degree to which it was skill-related imagery or anxiety management that contributed to the gains seen. Although this fact does not diminish the efficacy of the intervention for a group effect, it does hinder an interpretation of which component might be emphasized with athletes who appear to have performance decrements that principally originate in the planning or execution of complex skills more than in anxiety or tension. This seems important because recent sports research[59] suggests that progressive muscle relaxation (a somatic intervention) is more effective than cognitive approaches for managing anxiety among athletes. Also, a recent study[60] that combined VMBR with video-taped modeling of correct technique showed an increase in free-throw percentage among female collegiate basketball players, while no effects were seen for the progressive relaxation and imagery components of VMBR without observing the model.

KEY COMPONENTS

Imagery and goal setting are key components of many cognitive-behavioral interventions that originated in abnormal psychology and stress-management. Although clinical interventions have been adopted and modified for application with healthy athletes, it is informative to consider the usefulness of imagery and goal setting as independent performance aids. They might be equally as effective for most athletes as procedures founded in clinical methods, yet would not require clinical training. Also, studies on imagery and goal-setting in sport might help determine why (or if) cognitive-behavioral interventions can enhance sport performance in unique ways.

MENTAL PRACTICE

There is growing evidence from neurophysiological experiments and case studies, behavioral experiments on motor learning and control, and anecdotal self-reports by athletes that covert mental (symbolic) images or thoughts about movement are associated with the neuromuscular control of skilled-limb motion.[61] For example, complex movement patterns are reliably reproduced to precise locations when points on the supplementary pre-motor cortex (located anterior to the primary motor area and adjacent to the origin of thought) are stimulated.[62] Conversely, these movements are impaired when the pre-motor area is ablated. Electromyographic evidence confirms that intrinsic (mind's eye) thoughts of voluntary movement (without actual movement) produce subthreshold EMG activity, while extrinsic (as if a spectator) images of the same motion do not.[63] Moreover, it is firmly established across a wide range of movement speeds, amplitudes, durations, and periods of memory retention that movements are more accurately reproduced when the performer plans or pre-selects the location and degree of a limb motion than when this is constrained by an experimenter.[64] Finally, the time delay between the sensory reception of an environmental stimulus for motion and the elevation of muscle electrical-action potential (pre-motor period) increases in proportion to the complexity of the movement required; this indicates increased mental planning prior to execution. And a so-called readiness potential can be measured by surface electrodes along pre-central and parietal areas (along which motivated thought originates) of human scalp as early as 800 msec before even simple voluntary movements (e.g., finger flexion) begin.[62]

These findings have led to studies of the effectiveness of imagined (covert) rehearsal, or mental practice, as an adjunct or alternative to physical practice for enhancing skilled-motor performance.[40] The purported mechanisms underlying mental imagery essentially encompass either cognitive (abstract, symbolic) processes, whereby complex movements or movement situations are anticipated and appropriate responses are pre-planned, or somatic processes, whereby subthreshold innervation of the muscles involved in the motion somehow enhances their subsequent force or firing pattern during real-time execution.

Well over 100 studies of mental rehearsal and motor performance have been published, but their lack of uniformity has hindered interpretation. In their excellent meta-analysis of the mental practice literature, Feltz and Landers[65] recently proposed that mental practice effects (1) are primarily associated with cognitive-symbolic rather than motoric components of skills; (2) are found both in early and later stages of learning a skill (the stage may depend on whether the skill is predominantly cognitive, e.g., discrete and serial tasks like throwing, swinging, kicking, diving, rather than motoric, e.g., continuous or repetitive tasks like bicycling, running, swimming, dancing); (3) are probably not the results of sub-threshold innervation of the muscles to be used in the actual motion; and (4) may be the indirect result of optimizing physiological arousal and attentional focus for warm-up responses that can be generalized across many skills, e.g., metabolic arousal, or are specific to the demands of a particular skill, e.g., optimal muscle tension or concentration.

This analysis reveals several problems with the use of mental imagery as a psychological aid in sport. It is common for imagery interventions to employ a standard set of imagery-inducing instructions for all athletes on a sports team and for different sports. Yet the degree of symbolic control found in high-level skill varies widely. Even among athletes in the same sport and level of expertise, it is likely that there are significant differences in imaging abilities, and the need for symbolic control may vary substantially across small differences in technique. Although it is believed that as novices at a skill we all initially pass through a learning stage that is predominantly cognitive, this has less bearing on high levels of performance where acute ergogenic aids are a concern.

On the other hand, even in sports in which individual movements become automated, advanced skills often become behaviorally more complex in the sequencing and timing of component movements (e.g., diving, tumbling, apparatus) or in the reaction to a rapidly changing sport setting. In these instances it is likely that problem-solving or anticipation could benefit from covert rehearsal and pre-planning if the predictions an athlete makes about the sport environment or upcoming movements are improved in speed or accuracy. Mental errors could thus be identified and reduced.

It is important to note, however, that there are many aspects of motor skill plans that are likely never conscious. We learn to walk, run, throw, jump, kick, strike, and ride bicycles without "knowing" rules about how.

Though most of us can improve these basic skills if well taught, how much we can improve or to what degree gains are cognitive in origin remains unknown. Clearly, telling people how to move is often inadequate, and it is unclear to what degree observing or feeling proper technique is a mental rather than a perceptual event. Indeed, skilled athletes often are completely unaware of (or cannot verbalize) how they perform and, paradoxically, can even exacerbate a temporary technique problem by attempting to consciously control ballistic skills (where movement velocities exceed the known speed with which the nervous system can correct a movement error). Likewise, even though the vividness with which many athletes are able to image their technique may well reflect a memory of conjoint somathetic and motor processes (e.g., kinesthesia) which is important for the planning of a complex movement, this does not indicate that the image is formed apart from physical practice and knowledge of actual results. The mental image may be a side effect, not a cause, of physical skill.

There is less reason to expect that image-induced gains in muscle action potential will translate into skill enhancement. First, studies show that muscle innervation during imagery is not necessarily limited to the muscles involved in the imagined motion; localization may depend on movement experience with the motion or on concentration/relaxation skills. Most damaging to an innervation effect, however, are the apparent lack of proprioceptive feedback from the limb because no muscle contraction or joint movement occurs and the absence of knowledge of movement outcomes. Without a known mechanism for error detection (by comparing the planned or expected motor efference with the actual discharge and with resulting outcomes of actually executing the movement plan), it is not theoretically possible for motor learning to occur.[61, 64] It seems unreasonable that memory of the imagined efference would be sufficiently retained for later comparisons with a movement. It is more likely that the electromyographic recordings observed during an imagined complex movement are corollary discharges that reflect a memory of physical practice history rather than an independent mental skill.

When acute performance gains accompany imagery in principally noncognitive skills (e.g., weightlifting or sprinting), it seems more likely that they result indirectly from preparatory arousal or attention focusing (either might increase or regulate the number, rate, or sequence of muscle fiber recruitment) than directly from a symbolic change in cortical brain function. This is consistent with studies describing the mental preparation strategies used naturally by power athletes.[17] Characteristic strategies involve concentration and selective arousal, while preparation time increases as performance demands grow. Yet experimental attempts to teach (by cognitive means) these strategies to others or to alter an athlete's preferred strategy have not been encouraging.

GOAL SETTING

In a comprehensive review of goal setting and task performance across many environments and behaviors, Locke and colleagues[66] recently concluded that in 90 per cent of the studies between 1969 and 1980, specific quantitative goals that were challenging but attainable led to higher performance than did easy, more generalized qualitative (e.g., do your best) goals or no goals. This effect appeared independent of intrinsic personality factors related to goal striving such as self-esteem and achievement need (these factors, however, include and interact with goal setting). Goal-setting effects were optimized when motivation was as necessary as ability and when feedback about progress toward the goal and rewards for goal attainment were provided. Goals apparently affect performance by focusing attention on specific behaviors needed to produce outcomes (not just on the outcomes themselves), by energizing effort, by increasing persistence, and by providing incentives for the development by the individual of multiple or alternate plans to attain the same goal; these can be preferred by the person more than those initially provided.

Goal setting is a fundamental component of many cognitive-behavioral approaches to behavior modification. Common approaches involve identifying and specifying desired long-term or distant goals and the necessary direction and intensity of effort required to achieve them. This is typically accompanied by scheduling a sequence of prerequisite, step-up, or proximal goals that, if carried out, will ensure production of the final goal.

These approaches seem essential to establishing contest, season, and career motivation for strategic and peak execution of existing or developing sport skills. They exemplify a cognitive counterpart and possible complement to behavioristic approaches such as shaping. Goal-setting techniques seem particularly important in endurance or power sports where it is necessary to taper or cycle the volume of physical conditioning so that overuse injuries or staleness do not compromise peak expression of physiological capacities. Goal-setting techniques also appear critical to the assignment and acceptance of individual athlete's roles in a way that best enhances team goals. Likewise, they are useful for optimizing athletes' expectations about current and potential skill levels or outcome probabilities.

This latter use can be problematic, however, because it is often difficult to determine an athlete's ultimate potential skill and because competitive sport outcomes often depend on dynamic interactions between opponents within changing environments. Objective predictions are thus inexact; outcomes depend on more than personal effort. When projections are wrong, paradoxical performance outcomes can result from falsely retarded development of skill and inappropriate preparation or from misplaced frustration due to false expectations.

Despite the widespread use of goal setting by sport psychologists, coaches, and athletes, systematic studies of its effectiveness for sports (apart from its inclusion as part of cognitive-behavioral intervention packages) have not been reported. This is noteworthy because sport behaviors often are quite different from the industrial tasks studied in most goal setting research. Yet it is likely that when cognitive-behavioral interventions are effective with mentally healthy athletes, it is because of the instructional and motivating aspects of goal setting as much as the reduction of maladaptive thoughts and emotions.

CAVEATS

Because the influence of psychology on sport performance is often transient, it is difficult to measure in a precise and reproducible way. As a result, the predictive accuracy needed to show convincingly that a given intervention will produce a specific outcome for a particular athlete is a challenging scientific objective. The attainment of this goal has been hindered, however, because the strength of scientific inference found in published research varies widely from study to study. Current knowledge must be drawn from pre-experimental (uncontrolled case and group change or cross-sectional static group comparisons and correlations) and quasi-experimental (controlled time-series case studies or nonequivalent control group comparisons) investigations as well as from more interpretable controlled experiments (many, however, lack convincing placebo contrasts to discount generalized effects due more to the experimenter/therapist or to subject/client expectations).

Although potentially generalizable explanations for outcomes are suggested by many studies, the lack of uniformity in the type of subjects and sports, the performance-outcome measures employed, the psychological factors tested, and the specified procedures of the interventions make it difficult, if not impossible, to draw conclusions that are reliable and have external validity across interventions, sports, and athletes. There are few standardized principles to guide psychological aids in sport. In most instances it is best to view available studies as indicative of what can happen, not what will happen. For example, across all subjects and skills studied, the estimated performance effect of mental practice (one of the most widely studied and touted aids), is about one half of one standard deviation[65]; behaviorally robust effects usually exceed one standard deviation.

While it is established that selected personality traits can help predict a number of performance-related responses, based on intervention studies it is now possible only to specify an average effect for the group, not the effect on an individual. Certainly, some athletes respond in opposite ways to those predicted by the intervention, and many do not respond at all. Moreover, extraneous factors (many times unidentified) can operate in sport settings to influence performance or its determinants in ways different from the environments of controlled studies. Thus, knowing that a psychological factor *can* affect a performance outcome does not necessarily indicate that the factor can be *changed* in a feasible way or that a performance *gain will result* if the factor is changed.

PROFESSIONAL CAUTIONS

Despite these methodological concerns, the argument for an association between sport performance and controlled psychological events remains compelling for scientists, service providers, and discerning athletes and coaches.[67-69] Indeed, recognition of psychological events as potent influences on performance is reflected by the standard investigative procedure in pharmacological research of placebeo trials and experimenter blinding to control for subject expectancy effects. Reviews on the ergogenic effects of drugs, nutrition, caffeine, amphetamines, anabolic steroids, oxygen, and water and electrolytes pointedly mention that psychological factors can systematically contribute to or confound the predicted performance outcomes.[2, 70]

Recent acceleration of applied or professional use of psychological principles and techniques in sport has, however, met with legal, ethical, and academic controversies[71] over who (licensed psychologists, psychiatrists, physical educators, others) is qualified to offer services to athletes or coaches, what delivery model is most needed or most effective (educational, developmental, or therapeutic), and what the proven benefits and risks associated with current principles and technologies are. The growth in professional service has in part fueled interest in establishing an Exercise and Sports Psychology Division within the American Psychological Association (APA) as well as a membership debate within the academically oriented North American Society for the Psychology of Sport and Physical Activity (NASPSPA) that prompted the recent formation of a splinter group known as the Association for the Advancement of Applied Sport Psychology (AAASP). In addition, the United States Olympic Committee's Sports Psychology Registry was formed to provide quality control for professionals wishing to work with Olympic athletes. A peer-refereed list of sports psychologists with expertise in research, education, or clinical services is available for interested sports national governing bodies (NGB's). However, NGB's are not bound to use the registry, and such a registry cannot ensure competence for work with either Olympic caliber athletes or others.

The American College of Sports Medicine includes principles of human psychology and behavior change as learning objectives in its professional certifications for program director, exercise test technician, exercise specialist, and fitness leader but does not offer certifications for sports psychology. The American Alliance for Health, Physical Education, Recreation, and Dance, which includes the nation's largest professional physical education organization, has a Sport Psychology Academy but no designated certification for professional sport psychology services.

Because numerous medical or performance problems experienced by athletes can require or will benefit from psychological assessment and intervention, physicians or sports medicine teams who elect to include psychological methods as adjuncts or alternatives to care should be aware of their potential risks (e.g., clinical reactance by some clients to hypnosis[47] or relaxation techniques[72]; ineffective crisis screening and intervention) as well as their potential benefits. This is especially true in situations in which a nonlicensed sports psychology consultant might become involved with a problem having known or suspected clinical implications (e.g., depressive, phobic, panic, and psychotic disorders or life crises); an athlete's problems can frequently reflect mental health concerns that extend beyond sports settings, but these can be overlooked by an unqualified consultant. Likewise, insight into sports performance problems that can be clearly determined as subclinical may be best provided by a professional with extensive training in both human behavior and sport science. Analysis of sports skills requires equally specialized training.

CONCLUSION

Growing numbers of sports psychologists apparently assume that the psychological events associated with top sports performance are known and can be reliably changed in beneficial ways by existing psychological and behavioral techniques. Although the theories that underlie some of the popular interventions are persuasive, their techniques still are debated in general and clinical psychology. Present-day claims for success in sports exceed empirical data that satisfy conventional standards for internal (results are best attributable to the intervention) and external (results are reproducible with other athletes in other sports settings) validity.[73] This suggests that athletes and coaches will be as well served by future efforts to verify, refine, and create psychological techniques that can be effectively and predictably applied in sports as by present efforts to promote psychological applications in sports. Clinicians often justify scientific shortfalls by social validity (e.g., importance of the change and consumer/client satisfaction), but this does not permit conclusions about ergogenic effects that are specific to the principles of the intervention rather than to those that capitalize and depend upon client expectations or a general motivational effect. Nonspecific effects can often be used to good advantage by an artful clinician, but they are not enough upon which to base a profession.

In a recent synopsis of advances in sports medicine and exercise science during the preceding decade,[74] Carl Gisolfi (immediate past president of the American College of Sports Medicine) implied that the role of brain functions in exercise and sports performance remains a fruitful but poorly understood area of study and application. Although frustrating to the clinician, my review of the scholarly literature on psychological aids in sports yields the same diagnosis. Collectively, psychological interventions in sports appear better than no intervention when the athlete is healthy and there is clearly room for improvement; whether the performance gains observed are owing to the purported mechanisms of the intervention or to nonspecific motivating or enabling effects is unclear. Because most athletes are healthy and resilient, potential performance benefits seem to outweigh psychological or medical risks; in these cases psychological aids are, at worst, innocuous.

For some athletes, however, mental or physical health is the principal concern, while performance or behavior problems are superimposed. Clinical methods are indicated, and they can aid a return to normal function by first resolving the more important health problem. In such cases, the failure of an intervention, or at times the intervention itself, carries risks that are potentially great. For these reasons the use of psychological aids in sports should be preceded by a careful cost/benefit analysis that considers the subjective goals and appraisals and the well-being of the athlete in addition to the objective performance standards of the sport.

ACKNOWLEDGMENT: Thanks go to Julie Messer for preparing the manuscript.

REFERENCES

1. Dishman RK: Contemporary sport psychology. Exerc Sport Sci Rev 10: 120, 1982.
2. Morgan WP (ed): Ergogenic Aids and Muscular Performance. New York, Academic Press, 1972.
3. Landers DM: The arousal-performance relationship revisited. Res Q Exerc Sports 51:77, 1980.
4. Morgan WP: Psychogenic factors and exercise metabolism: A review. Med Sci Sports Exerc 17:309, 1985.
5. Massey BH, Johnson WR, Kramer GF: Effect of warm-up exercise upon muscular performance using hypnosis to control the psychological variable. Res Q Exerc Sport 32:63, 1960.
6. Ekman P, Levenson RW, Friesen WV: Autonomic nervous system activity distinguishes among emotions. Science 221:1208, 1983.
7. Schwartz GE, Weinberger D, Singer JA: Cardiovascular differentiation of happiness, sadness, anger and fear following imagery and exercise. J Psychosom Med 43:343, 1981.
8. Skubic E, Hilgendorf J: Anticipatory, exercise, and recovery heart rates of girls as affected by four running events. J Appl Physiol 19:853, 1964.
9. Berman R, Simonson E, Heron W: Electrocardiographic effects associated with hypnotic suggestion in normal and coronary sclerotic individuals. J Appl Physiol 7:89, 1954.
10. Morgan WP, Raven PB, Drinkwater BL, Horvath SM: Perceptual and metabolic responsivity to standard bicycle ergometry following various hypnotic suggestions. Int J Clin Exp Hypn 21:86, 1973.
11. Morgan WP, Hirota K, Weitz GA, et al: Hypnotic perturbation of perceived exertion: Ventilatory consequences. Am J Clin Hypn 18:182, 1976.
12. Benson H, Dryer T, Hartley LH: Decreased Vo_2 consumption during exercise with elicitation of the relaxation response. J Human Stress 4:38, 1978.
13. Gervino EV, Veazey AE: The physiologic effects of Benson's relaxation response during submaximal aerobic exercise. J Cardiac Rehabil 4:254, 1984.
14. Ziegler SG, Klinzing J, Williamson K: The effects of two stress management training programs on cardiorespiratory efficiency. J Sport Psychol 4:280, 1982.
15. Cavanaugh PR, Kram R: The efficiency of human movement—a statement of the problem. Med Sci Sports Exerc 17:304, 1985.

16. Ikai M, Steinhaus A: Some factors modifying the expression of human strength. J Appl Physiol 16:157, 1961.
17. Weinberg RS: The relationship between mental preparation strategies and motor performance: A review and critique. Quest 33:195, 1981.
18. Johnson WR, Kramer GF: Effects of stereotyped nonhypnotic, hypnotic, and posthypnotic suggestions upon strength, power, and endurance. Res Q Exerc Sport 32:522, 1961.
19. Morgan WP, Horstman DH, Cymerman A, et al: Facilitation of physical performance by means of a cognitive strategy. Cog Ther Res 7:251, 1983.
20. Dishman RK: Aerobic power, estimation of physical ability and attraction to physical activity. Res Q Exerc Sport 49:285, 1978.
21. Dishman RK, Holly RG, Schelegle E: Psychometric, perceptual, and metabolic predictors of self-limited maximal and submaximal treadmill performance. Med Sci Sports Exerc 17(2):198, 1985.
22. Lanning W: The privileged few: Special counseling needs of athletes. J Sport Psychol 4:19, 1982.
23. Nelson ES: The effects of career counseling on freshman college athletes. J Sport Psychol 4:32, 1982.
24. Cooker PG, Caffey CA: Addressing the cognitive and affective needs of college athletes: Effects of group counseling on self-esteem, reading skills, and coaches' perceptions of attitude. J Sport Psychol 6:377, 1984.
25. Wolpe J, Lazarus AA: Behavior Therapy Techniques. Elmsford, NY, Pergamon Press, 1966.
26. Wolpe J: Psychotherapy by Reciprocal Inhibition. Stanford, CA, Stanford University Press, 1958.
27. Woolfolk RL, Lehrer PM (eds): Principles and Practice of Stress Management. New York, Guilford Press, 1984.
28. Rushall BS, Siedentop D: The Development and Control of Behavior in Sport and Physical Education. Philadelphia, Lea and Febiger, 1972.
29. Dickinson JA: A Behavioral Analysis of Sport. Princeton, NJ, Princeton Book Company, 1977.
30. Martin GL, Hrycaiko D: Behavior Modification and Coaching: Princples, Procedures and Research. Springfield, IL, Charles C Thomas, 1983.
31. Donahue JA, Gillis JH, King K: Behavior modification in sport and physical education. J Sport Psychol 2:311, 1980.
32. Allison M, Ayllon T: Behavioral coaching in the development of skills in football, gymnastics, and tennis. J Appl Behav Anal 13:297, 1980.
33. Buzas H, Ayllon T: Differential reinforcement in coaching tennis skills. Behav Mod 5:372, 1981.
34. Shapiro ES, Shapiro S: Behavioral coaching in the development of skills in track. Behav Mod 9:211, 1985.
35. Roberts AH: Research, training, and clinical roles. Am Psychol 4:938, 1985.
36. Young LD, Blanchard EB: Awareness of heart activity and self-control of heart rate: A failure to replicate. Psychophysiology 21:361, 1984.
37. Dishman RK: Stress management procedures. In Williams M (ed): Ergogenic Aids in Sport. Champaign, IL, Human Kinetics Publishers, 1983.
38. Jacobson E: Progressive relaxation. Chicago, University of Chicago Press, 1938.
39. Antal LC, Good CS: The effects of oxprenolol on pistol shooting under stress. In Elsdon-Dew RW, Wink CAS, Birdwood GFB (eds): The Cardiovascular, Metabolic, and Psychological Interface. London, Royal Society of Medicine, Academic Press, 1979.
40. Silva JM: Covert rehearsal strategies. In Williams M (ed): Ergogenic Aids in Sport. Champaign, IL, Human Kinetics Publishers, 1983.
41. Kirschenbaum DS, Tomarken AJ: On facing the generalization problem: The study of self-regulatory failure. In Kendall PC (ed): Advances in Cognitive-Behavioral Research and Therapy. Vol 1. New York, Academic Press, 1982, p 119.
42. Ellis A: Reason and Emotion in Psychotherapy. New York, Lyle Stuart, 1962.

43. Beck A: Cognitive Therapy and Emotional Disorders. New York, International University Press, 1976.
44. Cautela JR, Wisocki PA: Thought-stopping procedure: Description, application, and learning theory interpretations. Psychol Rec 27:255, 1977.
45. Dishman RK: Medical psychology in exercise and sport. Med Clin North Am 69:123, 1985.
46. Meyers AW, Schleser R: A cognitive behavioral intervention for improving basketball performance. J Sport Psychol 2:69, 1980.
47. Morgan WP, Brown D: Hypnosis. In Williams M (ed): Ergogenic Aids in Sport. Champaign, IL, Human Kinetics Publishers, 1983.
48. Meichenbaum D: Cognitive Behavior Modification: An Integrative Approach. New York, Plenum Press, 1977.
49. Smith RE: Development of an integrated coping response through cognitive-affective stress management training. In Sarason IG, Spielberger CD (eds): Stress and Anxiety. Washington, DC, Hemisphere Publishing, 1980.
50. Benson HL: The Relaxation Response. New York, William Morrow and Company, 1975.
51. Mahoney MJ: Cognitive skills and athletic performance. In Kendall PC, Hollon SD (eds): Cognitive-Behavioral Interventions: Theory, Research and Procedures. New York, Academic Press, 1979, p 423.
52. Bandura A: Self-efficacy: Toward a unifying theory of behavioral change. Psychol Rev 84:191, 1977.
53. Rachman S (ed): Advances in Behavior Research and Therapy. Oxford, Pergamon Press, 1978, Vol 1.
54. Heyman SR: Comparisons of successful and unsuccessful competitors: A reconsideration of methodological questions and data. J Sport Psychol 4:295, 1982.
55. Feltz D: Path analysis of the causal elements in Bandura's theory of self-efficacy and an anxiety-based model of avoidance behavior. J Pers Soc Psychol 42:764, 1982.
56. Nideffer RM: The Ethics and Practice of Applied Sport Psychology. Ithaca, New York, Mouvement Publications, 1981.
57. Suinn RM: Imagery and Sports. In Sheikh AA (ed): Imagery: Current Theory, Research and Application. New York, John Wiley and Sons, 1983, p 507.
58. Seabourne TG, Weinberg RS, Jackson A, et al: Effect of individualized, nonindividualized, and package intervention strategies on karate performance. J Sport Psychol 7:40, 1985.
59. Hatfield BD, Landers DM: Psychophysiology—a new direction for sport psychology. J Sport Psychol 5:243, 1983.
60. Hall EG, Erffmeyer ES: The effect of visuo-motor behavior rehearsal with videotaped modeling on free throw accuracy of intercollegiate female basketball players. J Sport Psychol 5:343, 1983.
61. Schmidt RA: Motor Control and Learning. Champaign, IL, Human Kinetics Publishers, 1982.
62. Henatsch HD, Langer HH: Basic neurophysiology of motor skills in sport: A review. Int J Sports Med 6:2, 1985.
63. Jacobson E: Electrical measurements of neuromuscular states during mental activities. Am J Physiol 96:115, 1931.
64. Stelmach GE (ed): Information Processing in Motor Control and Learning. New York, Academic Press, 1978.
65. Feltz DL, Landers DM: The effects of mental practice on motor skill learning and performance: A meta-analysis. J Sport Psychol 5:25, 1983.
66. Locke EA, Saari LM, Shaw KN, et al: Goal setting and task performance 1969–1980. Psychol Bull 90:125, 1981.
67. Nideffer RM: Applied sport psychology. In Strauss RH (ed): Sports Medicine. Philadelphia, W.B. Saunders Company, 1984, p 501.
68. Browne MA, Mahoney MJ: Sport psychology. Ann Rev Psychol 35:605, 1984.
69. Straub WF, Williams JM: Cognitive Sport Psychology. Lansing, NY, Sport Science Associates, 1984.

70. Williams MH (ed): Ergogenic Aids in Sport. Champaign, IL, Human Kinetics Publishers, 1983.
71. Dishman RK: Identity crises in North American sport psychology: Academics in professional issues. J Sport Psychol 5:123, 1983.
72. Heide FJ, Borkovec TD: Relaxation-induced anxiety: Mechanisms and theoretical implications. Behav Res Ther 22:1, 1984.
73. Campbell DT, Stanley JC: Experimental and Quasiexperimental Designs for Research. Chicago, Rand McNally, 1963.
74. Legwold G, Moore M, Hage P: Sports medicine: The momentum continues. Phys Sportsmed 11(6):152, 1983.

10

WHY ARE SPORTS RECORDS IMPROVING?

PER-OLOF ÅSTRAND, M.D.
ANDERS BORGSTROM

> The ultimate object of all athletic records is to set down the best results that men have brought about, severally, and together, in public matches under well-established conditions, governed by rules and competent judges. Ideally, one thereby learns what is the most men have been able so far to achieve through the agency of matured, trained bodies. The records in which we are most interested tell us the limits beyond which no one has yet been able to go.
>
> P. WEISS[1]

Why have the records of sports performance improved? Several factors, which vary in importance depending on the characteristics of the sport, must be considered. The following factors will be discussed in detail:

—Selection from a larger and healthier population

—Better training methods and preparation

—Improved techniques

—Improved materials

—Psychological aspects

—Scientific support

—Doping

—Physiological aspects

This discussion will choose examples mainly from track and field events. Figures 10–1 to 10–6 illustrate the development of world records in several sports from the beginning of this century, when systematic documentation of the world's best performances started. For evident reasons, one can trace the effects of two world wars in the statistics—there is a retardation in progress during, and for some years after, the wars.

SELECTION FROM A LARGER AND HEALTHIER POPULATION

More and more individuals, particularly women, are attracted by sports activities. More and more nations are represented in the sports arena. As preventive and curative health measures become more successful throughout the Third World, millions of teenagers will, hopefully, have a chance to enjoy sports. These factors make it more likely that individuals with talent for a special sport will be noticed by the experts.

BETTER TRAINING METHODS AND PREPARATION

Training volume has increased and training methods have improved dramatically. Today, top athletes are not "true amateurs" as in the days when the Olympic oath included the statement that athletes did not compete for improvement of their economy. Certainly, top athletes have always managed to make money on their sport, but today this is permissible and can involve large amounts of money. In other words, athletes can now devote more time to training and can train year-round in a climate that is optimal.

IMPROVED TECHNIQUES

In some events, changes in the rules have made a development of the technique possible. In the early rules for high jump it was stated that when passing the crossbar (1) the jumper's buttocks should be on a lower level than his or her head, and (2) the feet should be before the head. However, in 1936 the rules were changed, and the only restriction was that the take-off be accomplished from one foot. Until then the scissors style had dominated. However, the "western roll," actually introduced by Horine in 1910, gave H.M. Osborne the gold medal in the 1924 Olympic Games, but the judges had great problems deciding whether or not his jumping style conformed to the rules. Probably this and other similar incidents made it necessary to change the rules. Dick Fosbury's victory with his "flop style" in the 1968 Olympic Games introduced in a spectacular way today's dominant technique.

Covering the circle for the shot put, discus, and hammer throw with rubber material or concrete facilitated the development of new techniques.

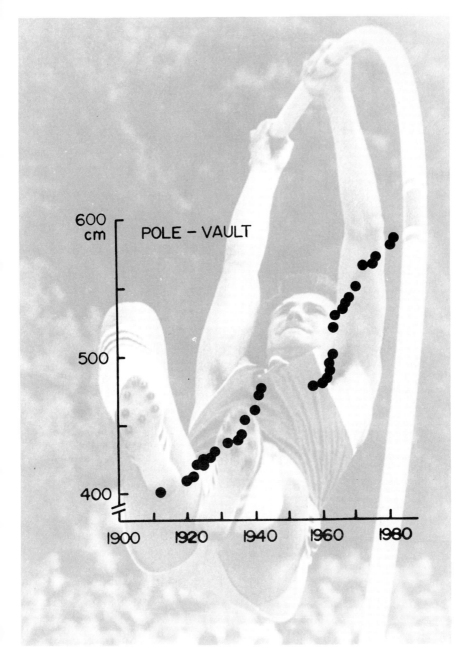

Figure 10–1. In 1960, Don Bragg broke the world record by jumping 480 cm with his steel pole. In 1961, the first record was set using a fiberglass pole (483 cm), and two years later John Pennel jumped 520 cm. The fiberglass pole effectively stores some of the athlete's energy developed during the run and, with good technique, that energy can be utilized at exactly the right moment. During the last 20 years, this catapult pole has changed very little in quality. Therefore, the continuously improved records must be due to better skill of the record breakers. Without the development of foam rubber mats on which to land, jumping with fiberglass poles would be dangerous. (Photograph: Sergei Bubka of the Soviet Union sets a new world record by jumping 588 cm in Saint-Denis Stadium, 1984. (Dagens Nyheter; Pressens Bild AB.)

149

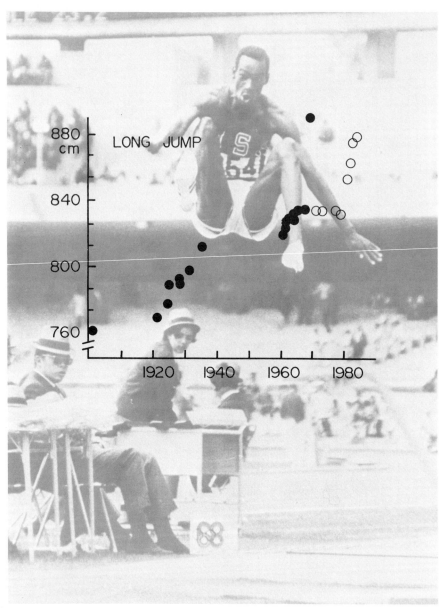

Figure 10–2. Bob Beamon's meteoric jump, sending him 890 cm from the take-off point in the Mexico City Olympic Games, was spectacular. "No other world track and field record excels the previous best performance by a comparable margin . . . Beamon's feat outshines all others. It is unlikely that the 8.90-meter record will ever be beaten" (Ernst Jokl). The unfilled circles denote the best results achieved during the years following 1968. Carl Lewis is gradually coming closer. If he had jumped his 879-cm leap at high altitude, assisted by a 2.00 m • s^{+1} wind against his back, Beamon's leap "into the next millennium" could have been surpassed. (Photograph: Bob Beamon in his 890-cm jump in the Olympic Games in Mexico City, 1968. (Pressens Bild AB.)

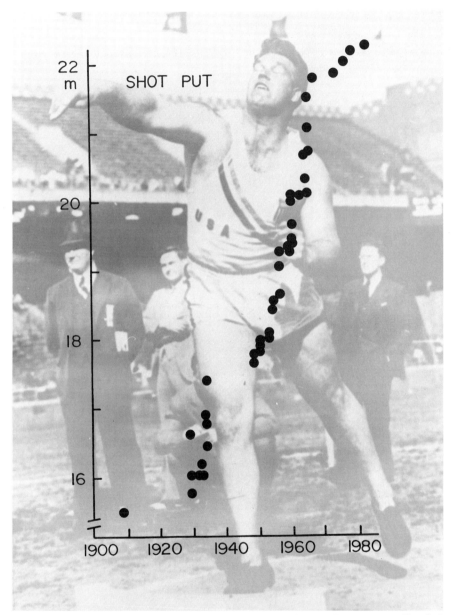

Figure 10–3. When the shot put event was young, it was predominantly a one-arm affair. Jack Torrance put the shot up on the finger tips and could thereby add extra power from the wrist. He reached a "phenomenal" 17.40 m in 1934, a result that survived attacks until 1948 (with World War II as a restriction in between). Parry O'Brien, in particular, introduced a new technique—starting in a low position with the back facing the direction of throw. The strength of leg and trunk muscles became more important, and it was logical that more strength training was included in preparation for the competitive season. O'Brien dominated the scene from 1953 until his last record noted in 1959. At the beginning of the 1950's the cinders in the ring were replaced by concrete, which facilitated the introduction of new techniques. In the mid 1970's, some shot putters launched a rotation to initiate the put. As mentioned in the text, there is a trend toward stagnation in the breaking of records during the last 20 years despite the growing popularity of the use of anabolic steroids. (Photograph: Jack Torrance, USA. (Pressens Bild AB.)

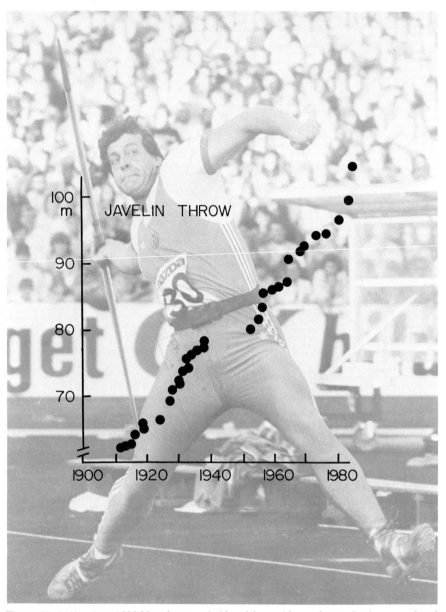

Figure 10–4. Already in 1932 Matti Järvinen, holder of the world record in javelin throw, predicted that someone one day would throw the javelin farther than 100 meters. His record at that time did not pass the 75-meter mark. In 1984 Uwe Hohn (GDR) hit the 104.80-meter point. There has been a dramatic development of the aerodynamic characteristics of the javelin over the years, with Frank Held (USA) as a pioneer. (He broke the world record in 1953 and again in 1955.) Held threw a specially designed javelin some 4 meters farther than traditional equipment, but this design was not approved by the authorities. One problem is to combine the javelin's aerodynamic ability to "float" on the air with a landing on its tip in accordance with the rules.

Legend continued on opposite page

IMPROVED MATERIALS

Technological innovations have played an important role in the performance explosion in many events.

The introduction of artificial surface on tracks improved conditions and, most importantly, maintained good lane conditions throughout a competition. Previously, the inner lane of track often became miserable as more and more feet wore it. The Pan-American Games in 1967 were the first big events to be held on an artificial surface. The modern materials on the thrower's circle also provided long-lasting and equal conditions for all competitors.

When starting blocks were permitted, the start in sprint events became faster.

The introduction of the fiberglass pole improved world records in pole vault in the 1960's. This is well illustrated in Figure 10–1. Actually, such a pole had been tried during the latter part of the 1950's, and an American, Alburley Dooley, was a pioneer in the development of a technique that efficiently utilized the elastic properties of the pole.

Without the foam rubber mat, the landing after a high jump and pole-vault jump would be hazardous. Actually, without this equipment the "flop style" and fiberglass pole would be dangerous to use.

The aerodynamic properties of the javelin and discus have been improved. The long throws, as illustrated in Figure 10–4, can be a threat to spectators. Also, it is often difficult to judge whether or not the javelin hits the ground with its point first. In 1986 a rule was passed which introduced a new javelin model with different aerodynamic characteristics than the traditional model. It is estimated that Hohn's world record (104.8 meters) is equivalent to approximately an 85-meter throw with the new model. The length-reducing effect is less pronounced with shorter throws. An "old" 90-meter mark would now be comparable to approximately 78 meters, and 60 meters to 59 meters. There is some sort of badminton ball effect. In addition, there is a much better chance that the javelin makes a "happy landing" on its point. It is unique that rules and equipment are introduced which reduce the performance as evaluated in meters.

When the breast stroke in swimming was modified to increase speed, a new event was born—the butterfly. Both styles are energetically expen-

---

The javelin throw is more effective with an extreme "bow" of the body before the throw. Actually already Järvinen applied this "bow." Stretched muscles can develop more strength than muscles at a shorter initial length. The javelin throw is, however, anatomically very demanding, and most throwers suffer from orthopedic problems, particularly in the elbow, at one or several stages of their career. As a curiosity it can be mentioned that the champion discus thrower Adolfo Consolini is reported to have given the javelin a 14-meter flight with the forbidden "soap style" (see text). (Photograph: Uwe Hohn, East Germany, throwing the javelin 104.80 meters. (Pressens Bild AB.)

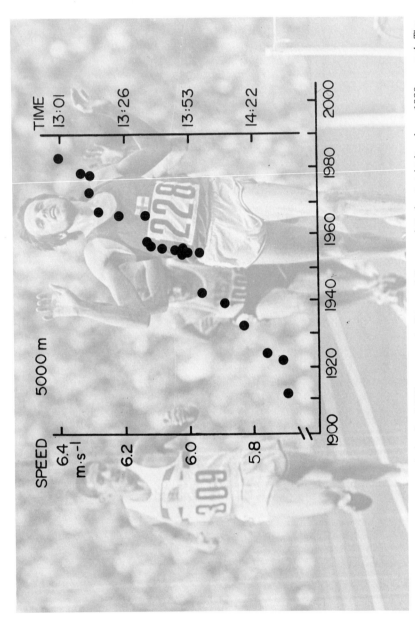

Figure 10–5. The world records for the 5,000-meter track distance follow a relatively straight line from 1920 onward. The introduction of the artificial surface on the lanes did not noticeably improve the records. An extrapolation to the world record for the year 2000 is tempting. (Photograph: Lasse Virén, Finland, wins the 5,000-meter race in the Olympic Games in Munich, 1972. (Pressens Bild AB.)

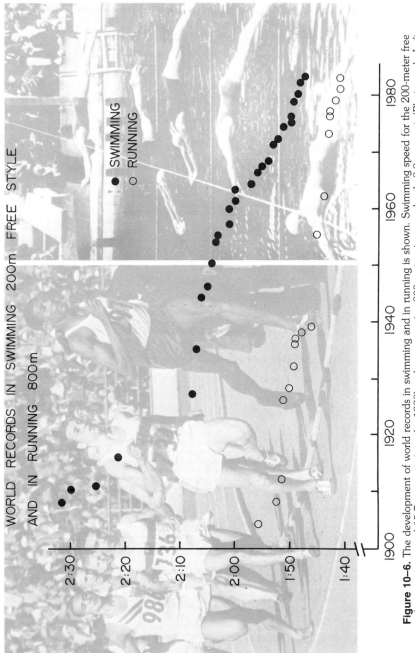

Figure 10–6. The development of world records in swimming and in running is shown. Swimming speed for the 200-meter free style event improved 15.7 per cent since the 1920's, whereas running 800 meters improved only 8.8 per cent. (Photograph: Left panel: Arthur Wint, Jamaica, is leading in the final 800-meter race in the 1952 Olympics in Helsinki. No. 734—Ulzheimer, Germany; 736—Steines, Germany; 986—Whitfield, USA, the winner. (UPI Photo; Pressens Bild AB.)

155

sive, so it is realistic that the longest distance swum in competition is 200 meters.

Some techniques have been prohibited for safety reasons, namely climbing on the pole in pole vault and a somersault in the long jump. In Spain the technique in a traditional sport was adopted for the javelin throw. The thrower initiates the throw with fast rotations, and the back part of the javelin is prepared with soap to reduce the friction against the palm when the javelin glides out of the hand. For evident reasons, this "soap style" is forbidden.

PSYCHOLOGICAL ASPECTS

Good performance depends on expectation, which in part determines tactics. With a world record of 3 minutes 30 seconds in the 1500 meter run, the goal may be to run in 3:29, but not in 3:20! In some events there are no barriers, e.g., one does not know the limits. A perfect example is Bob Beamon's 890 cm aerial trip in the long jump in 1968. That jump improved in a snap the world record by 55 cm (Fig. 10–2). A parallel: At that time the world record in high jump was 228 cm. Who would have dreamed of putting the crossbar up to 240 cm, which would have, if successfully passed, resulted in a similar improvement in statistics?

From a psychological viewpoint, it is often a handicap to run in front of the pack for most of a 1500 meter race. The drawback has at least partly a physiological background: Even if there is no wind, the speed as such causes significant air resistance. Running behind another competitor in a "shielded" position can save 4 to 6 per cent of the energy cost.[2] From both a psychological and a physiological aspect, an even speed throughout the race up to the final spurt usually gives the best time.

SCIENTIFIC SUPPORT

It is difficult to prove to what extent medical science has helped athletes in their pursuit of new records. Often the athletes have been one step ahead, applying trial-and-error methods, followed by the physiologists whose studies have revealed mechanisms that can explain why a particular regimen can enhance performance. However, basic research from the 1930's and 1940's, confirmed in more recent studies, has proven that diet and fluid balance can affect physical performance decisively. As early as 1939, Christensen and Hansen reported that a carbohydrate-rich diet improved endurance in heavy exercise and that training could have a glycogen-saving effect that enhances aerobic capacity.[3]

Scientific data supported the belief in beneficial effects of a warm-up before high-intensity exercise.

Unfortunately, many athletes are injured during training and competition. Physicians and physical therapists try, often successfully, to get the athlete back to the arena as quickly as possible. Methods for treatment and rehabilitation are examined critically. If successful, they are then available for everyone.

DOPING

It is a tragedy that so many athletes, coaches, and physicians violate the rules in their ambitions to win and break world records. In this book many aspects of the doping problem are discussed. It is our personal belief that performance in few disciplines can be improved by pills beyond what the athlete can achieve through will power and stimulation from a cheering crowd. Actually, without doping he or she usually performs better. It seems, however, that many coaches and athletes are willing to adopt, uncritically, new concepts claimed to improve athletic performance.

It is interesting that the world record in shot put only increased from 21.78 meters in the mid 1960's to 22.02 meters in 1982. (It is now 22.22 meters. See Figure 10–3.) During that period the intake of anabolic steroids increased dramatically and probably involved many world-class shot putters. It is tempting to conclude that the intake or injection of such hormones has not contributed significantly to the world record statistics in shot put.

PHYSIOLOGICAL ASPECTS

Are the athletes of today superior in their physiological potential as compared with their ancestors? A high *maximal-oxygen uptake, or aerobic power*, is essential for success in sports utilizing large muscle groups in all-out efforts for several minutes or longer. In activities in which the body weight is carried, this aerobic power is related to body weight (oxygen uptake in $ml \cdot kg^{-1} \cdot min^{-1}$). However, in such exercises as rowing and swimming, oxygen uptake is given in $liters \cdot min^{-1}$. In 1937, Robinson et al.[4] reported that Don Lash, who held the world record for the two-mile race, attained a maximal oxygen uptake of 81.5 $ml \cdot kg^{-1} \cdot min^{-1}$ when running on the treadmill. Today, competitors have similar values recorded, but they run faster. (Lash's record was 8:58.4; today the best time recorded is 8:13.8.) This fact is intriguing. Evidently modern training principles allow the athlete to exercise at or closer to maximal aerobic power for longer periods of time. Another reason for improved performance is a higher power and capacity of the anaerobic (without oxygen) metabolic pathways (see below).

Better shoes and tracks cannot explain the superiority of modern athletes. Ronald Clark's 27:39.4 for 10,000 meters on a cinder track (1965) is not far from Henry Rono's 27:22.5 on an artificial surface (1978). For the 100-meter distance James Hines' time of 10.03 seconds on a cinder lane at sea level is not significantly slower than his time of 9.95 seconds when running on artificial surface the same year but at high altitude, which favors the sprinter because air resistance is reduced. The better results noted on distances demanding a high maximal oxygen uptake cannot be explained by better tracks and lanes.

There is a personal limit for maximal oxygen uptake. One example: A Swedish cross-country skier who in 1955 had just qualified for the national team had at that time a maximal oxygen uptake of 5.48 liters $\cdot$ min^{-1}. In 1963 it was about the same (5.60 liters $\cdot$ min^{-1}), but he had trained almost daily during the intervening eight years and had successfully participated in two Olympic Games and two world championships, winning several gold medals. In repeated tests, another skier never exceeded 5.88 liters $\cdot$ min^{-1} in maximal oxygen uptake, measured in 1955. He trained intensively and competed successfully until 1964, winning a gold medal in the 50-kilometer race in that year's Olympic Games.[5] There are few data from longitudinal studies of top athletes in running disciplines. There are indications that running times improve despite a stagnation in the maximal aerobic power. A slight improvement in running economy and the ability to run faster before a continuous accumulation of lactate sets in can be effects of the training.[5]

We have no methods available for an exact measurement of an individual's maximal *anaerobic* power and capacity. Therefore we do not know whether athletes of today have better anaerobic metabolism to support the contractile machinery of exercising muscles than did earlier generations of athletes. An increase in blood lactate concentration reflects a breakdown of glycogen in muscle. However, one cannot calculate from blood concentration how much lactate is produced. It is interesting to note that this lactate concentration is usually higher if measured after an important competition than after an all-out test in the laboratory. The tolerance for high lactate values and low pH apparently can be modified by psychological factors. It is remarkable that the pH in the arterial blood can fall below 7.0 after repeated one-minute maximal runs. A comparison of peak blood lactate concentrations after maximal physical performance in the laboratory or in connection with competition in top athletes does not indicate any differences over the last 30 years.

There is a continuous increase in body height (H) in most developed countries. Assuming a proportional increase in all dimensions, *maximal strength*, related to the surface area of the muscles, should be proportional to H^2 and *maximal work* and *torque*, which can be developed to H^3. The mean height on the participants in the decathlon in the Rome Olympic Games in 1960 was 184 cm. Approximately 30 years earlier the average height was 176 cm. These athletes' heights compare as the ratio 1.045:1, their muscle strength as 1.09:1, and work or torque as 1.14:1. Therefore, owing to different dimensions, the 4.5 per cent taller decathlon athlete can be expected to be 9 per cent stronger and to have the capacity to do 14 per cent more work than his shorter competitor. These advantages are particularly evident in such events as throwing the javelin and discus and putting the shot. Extrapolating these data to the development of world records in shot put, similar changes in body dimensions alone could explain a gain from 16 meters in 1930 to approximately 18 meters in 1960. But that year the shot was put 20 meters. No doubt, in sports in which body size will influence the results, the competitors, from a democratic point of view, should be classified according to weight as in boxing, wrestling, and weightlifting. Such classifications would, however, be unrealistic in track and field events!

SEXUAL DIMORPHISM

Table 10–1 compares world records for women and men. In swimming, the highest speeds attained by women are, on the average, 91.7 per cent of those reached by men. In track, women are relatively slower, with top speeds at the 90.0 per cent level. Actually, female swimmers have a better efficiency than male swimmers when swimming at a given speed. Different body composition and "design" can explain this finding.[6] In speed skating, women reach 91.8 per cent of men's world record speeds. In bicycling the percentage is 88.2 per cent. Perhaps a number of women with talent for bicycling have not yet discovered this discipline.

The largest difference in world records in track and field events between women and men is noticed in high jump, with the women's

TABLE 10–1. Women's World Records Compared with Those for Men

Track and Field			Swimming	
100 m	92.3		Freestyle	
200	90.8		100 m	90.1
400	91.4		200	91.2
800	89.8		400	92.7
1500	90.7		800	93.6
5000	86.8		1500	92.7
10000	87.2			
Marathon	90.1		Breast stroke	
4 × 100 m	91.1		100 m	90.2
4 × 400 m	89.9		200	92.9
High jump	86.6			
Long jump	83.5		Butterfly	
Speed Skating			100 m	91.6
500 m	92.1		200	92.9
1000	91.5			
1500	92.1		Back stroke	
3000	93.3		100 m	91.1
5000	90.0		200	91.1
Bicycling				
5 km	87.3		Medley	
10	87.8		200 m	92.2
20	89.6		400	93.2

From a selection of world records at the end of 1984. The women's times (speeds) are given as percentages of the men's records (= 100 per cent). In jumping, a similar calculation is done.

crossbar reaching 86.6 per cent of the men's 239 cm, and in long jump, in which the best woman jumped 83.5 per cent of Beamon's 890 cm. We have no explanation of why women are particularly "inferior" in jumping.

It is interesting to follow the progress in results for women and men over the years. In 1950 the highest speed during the 100-meter run for women was 88.7 per cent of the best male performance (92.3 per cent today). In 1950 in the 800-meter race the percentage speed was 80.2. Few women competed over longer distances even though the 800-meter race appeared in the Olympic Games as early as 1928. In high jump, the women's record was 81 per cent of the men's best result in 1950, 83 per cent in 1960, 84 per cent in 1970 and, as mentioned, close to 87 per cent in 1984. In long jump the figures are 77, 78, 77, and 83.5 per cent, respectively. The women's records have gradually crept closer to the men's levels. There are speculations, which have gained world-wide interest in the mass media, that women will sooner or later catch up to the men's world records, sooner in the marathon than in other events. We do not think so. There are basic, genetically-fixed sexual differences that are decisive for physical performance demanding muscular strength and high aerobic power. There are no physiological data indicating that women have a particularly high potential for long distance events such as the marathon race.

WORLD RECORDS IN SWIMMING AS COMPARED WITH RUNNING

It seems that swimming is the discipline that has the world record for breaking world records. During the Munich Olympic Games the swimming competitors produced 30 world records in 29 events. There are claims that swimming is still a developing discipline. Figure 10–6 illustrates the advances in 200-meter freestyle and 800-meter running since the turn of the century. The reason for selecting those events is that the present world records are not far from each other with regard to the times involved. Records in running can survive for years, but in swimming the records since 1950 have been broken often. One factor to consider is that the percentage increase in the number of pools over the years surpasses the number of new tracks. Specific training of muscular strength and flexibility may improve the swimming performance more than the running ability.

ALTITUDE TRAINING

Is training at high altitude beneficial for the oxygen transport system? Björn Ekblom discusses this in Chapter 4. The reason for bringing up this question here is that a study of the improvement of world records can enlighten the discussion. Acclimatization to high altitude is essential in the preparation for optimal performance in events demanding high aerobic power if the competition takes place at high altitude. Actually, the Olympic Games in Mexico City were not the first challenge forced upon the athletes to face new environmental conditions. In the winter Olympic Games in Squaw Valley in 1960, the athletes had to gasp at an altitude of approximately 2,000 meters (6,600 feet). Now to the point: It is a common belief that training at high altitude will also enhance the performance at lower altitudes. The history of world records does not support this hypothesis. In the years 1966, 1967, and particularly in 1968, the cream of the world's athletes spent long periods of time in Mexico City or at similar altitudes. Many scientific studies were conducted on these athletes. However, few world records in middle- and long-distance running were broken in those years. Nor in swimming were there any spectacular new records. New records would be expected at sea level if a sojourn at high altitude elicited an additional improvement of maximal aerobic power and endurance. In fact, in 1968, when certainly all Olympic candidates were extremely well-prepared, there were no new world records in middle- and long-distance running.

THE RECORD

Eric Segal[7] writes:

But without any question, the most famous barrier in sports history was the four minute mile. And yet I seriously wonder if it would have acquired such mystique if the first man to break it had not been that eloquent obsessive, Roger Bannister. Anyone who reads his autobiography cannot help but sense what an all-consuming fixation it was for him to run merely two seconds faster than he ever had before. After all, Glenn Cunningham, that great miler of the 1930's, claimed that he had often run better than four minutes in practice sessions, but it had never seemed important to do so officially in a race. He had just wanted to win.

Not Bannister. To him, breaking four minutes for the mile would be extending the "ultimate" in human capability. Indeed, *as a doctor* Bannister believed that the effort required would be so enormous that the runner would expend his entire oxygen reserve a few yards *before* the finish and have to complete the race as a semiconscious reflex action. He planned his race according to his own theories. The rest is history.

The photos of Bannister after his epoch-making run on May 6, 1954, show a totally exhausted man who by dint of courage and scientific preparation systematically depleted himself of *all* his resources to surpass all previous limits. His face shows that his body had not an ounce in reserve. He could not have done an instant better. The ultimate time for the mile had to be 3:59.4.

This was, I repeat, May 6, 1954. And yet on August 7 of the same year, Bannister ran 3:58.8—without collapsing.

Parodoxically, running a mile even faster proved to be less exhausting.

Because once he had surpassed the four-minute "limit," there was no magic in 3:58. Nor did there appear to be in 3:50. Values are what they are, Hamlet tells us, "because thinking makes it so."

On July 18, 1979, the London *Daily Express* wrote the following: "Coe came up to the final straight looking almost relaxed, hardly gasping . . . what a fantastic contrast to the complete exhaustion of . . . Sir Roger Bannister."

The limits are, of course, purely mental. Sebastian Coe was so relaxed in Oslo because he did not consider 3:49 any kind of ultimate. And when he finally begins to think in these terms, some mad idealist will appear in track shoes and prove him wrong. There are simply no absolute limits.

As Swedes we like to remember the comments of two runners who broke many world records in middle-distance running in the 1940's, Gunder Hägg and Arne Andersson: First of all, one mile is not a Swedish distance; secondly, the goal is to win, not to make spectacular times.

CONCLUSION

Many factors have contributed to improvements in sports world records. The complexities of the disciplines are decisive for the quantitative impact of the various factors. Probably the basic endowment of the human being has been most stable. Changes in training methods, tactics, techniques, rules, equipment, material, economy, an increase in the number of people engaged in sports—all of these factors have contributed to the improvements. Most likely it will be many years before we can write the final history of all world records, records that will never be surpassed. In some events one can see a retardation in the curves, in others not. As mentioned previously, in the javelin event it will be very difficult to beat Hohn's record owing to equipment modifications. In certain disciplines not discussed here one can, with great confidence, say that "this record can never be improved." One such discipline is shooting. With all bullets awarded 10 points, present rules do not permit a better achievement.

It should be emphasized that sports that cannot be evaluated by world records also are very popular with participants and spectators: racket sports, American football, cricket, soccer, gymnastics, and golf, just to mention a few. Beating a world record is not an essential stimulus for action.

ACKNOWLEDGMENT: Many thanks to Mr. A. Lennart Julin for valuable information.

REFERENCES

1. Pabst U (ed): Baden-Baden Report: The Limits of Sports. 11th Olympic Congress, 1981. Nationales Olympisches Komitee für Deutschland, D-8000 München 40, Western Germany, 1980.

2. Åstrand PO, Rodahl K: Applied sports physiology. In Textbook of Work Physiology, 3rd ed. New York, McGraw-Hill, 1986, Ch. 14.
3. Christensen EH, Hansen O: Arbeitsfähigkeit und Ehrnährung. Skand Arch Physiol 81:160, 1939.
4. Robinson S, Edwards HT, Dill DB: New records in human power. Science 85:409, 1937.
5. Åstrand PO, Rodahl K.: Physical training. In Textbook of Work Physiology, 3rd ed. New York, McGraw-Hill, 1986, Ch. 10.
6. Holmer I: Energy cost of arm stroke, leg kick, and the whole stroke in competitive swimming styles. Eur J Applied Physiol 33:105, 1974.
7. Segal E: Reflections on the right to one's own limit. In Pabst U (ed): Baden-Baden Report: the Limits of Sports. 11th Olympic Congress, 1981. Nationales Olympisches Komitee für Deutschland, D-8000 München 40, Western Germany, 1980.

II

THERAPEUTIC DRUGS

11

EFFECTS OF THERAPEUTIC DRUGS ON SPORTS PERFORMANCE

RICHARD H. STRAUSS, M.D.

Medications are used in the treatment of disease and injury among athletes much as they are used among nonathletes. The question often arises: "What effects do the drugs themselves, apart from the problem being treated, have on the athlete's performance in sports?" This question is addressed below.

In practice, the problem for which the athlete sees the physician has often already impaired his or her performance and requires treatment. Thus, a drug that has the side effect of temporarily impairing performance may be the best choice. However, if competition is imminent, the physician may wish to consider alternative treatments that do not further impair performance. Drugs are grouped below by therapeutic category in alphabetical order.

ALLERGY RELIEF (See under Antihistamines.)

ANABOLIC-ANDROGENIC STEROID HORMONES

These drugs may enhance muscular strength under some circumstances but have significant adverse effects (see Chapter 5). Their use by athletes is considered unethical and they are banned by many organizations.

ANALGESICS (See also under Anti-inflammatory Agents.)

Aspirin and acetaminophen apparently do not impair performance. The narcotics such as codeine are known to impair mental and physical

167

performance owing to central nervous system depression (see Chapter 7). Their use is banned by the International Olympic Committee.

ANOREXICS

Most appetite suppressants are stimulants. The use of stimulants in attempts to improve performance is discussed in Chapter 6. Many, particularly the amphetamines and sympathomimetics, are banned in international and national competition (see Chapter 8). Overstimulation can impair performance in sports in which judgment or fine motor control is required, such as gymnastics.

ANTACIDS

Generally, there is no effect on performance. The use of bicarbonate in attempts to improve endurance is discussed in Chapter 3. Constipation or diarrhea occasionally results from the use of antacids. (See also below under Histamine H_2 Receptor Antagonists.)

ANTIASTHMA

Albuterol, a beta$_2$-adrenergic bronchodilator, is particularly useful by inhalation for the prevention or treatment of exercise-induced asthma.[1] It has a slight stimulant effect but probably does not affect performance except that a mild tremor of the hands may be noted, which is unwanted in the shooting sports. Oral theophylline is useful in the long-term control of asthma. An inhaled corticosteroid sometimes is added. The above drugs can be used at the Olympic level, but most sympatho-mimetics are banned (see Chapter 8). The barbiturates that are included in some oral drug combinations for the treatment of asthma can impair performance.

ANTIBIOTICS

These generally have no effect on performance.[2, 3]

ANTICONVULSANTS

Because of their effects on the brain, anticonvulsants have a potential for impairing performance. In practice, many athletes have performed well while under careful treatment with anticonvulsants.

ANTIDEPRESSANTS

Occasionally, these drugs have been used by athletes in search of a stimulant effect or to improve concentration. Such use is not recommended. Although mood elevation may occur in normal persons with the monoamine oxidase (MAO) inhibitors, the tricyclic antidepressants usually act as sedatives.

ANTIDIABETIC AGENTS

Good control of diabetes is necessary for an individual to perform optimally. These agents do not improve performance beyond normal.

Owing to increased blood flow, insulin is absorbed more rapidly from its site of injection when that part of the body is exercised. Exercise tends to decrease the insulin requirement.[4]

ANTIDIARRHEALS

Drugs such as diphenoxylate and, to a lesser extent, loperamide have the potential for decreasing athletic performance due to a mild sedative effect. Bismuth subsalicylate does not sedate.

ANTIFUNGAL AGENTS

Topical antifungal agents are poorly absorbed and have no effect on performance.

ANTIHISTAMINES

Most of these drugs act as mild sedatives. Antihistamines are widely used in the treatment of colds and allergies as prescription and nonprescription medications and require a word of caution. Athletes should avoid taking them prior to a contest in which top performance is necessary. In addition, antihistamines should be avoided even during practice in those sports, such as springboard diving and gymnastics, in which an error in judgment or timing can result in injury to the participant. In scuba diving, antihistamines may act synergistically with nitrogen narcosis to further impair judgment underwater.

ANTI-INFLAMMATORY AGENTS

The nonsteroidal anti-inflammatory drugs generally do not impair performance. Occasional users complain of subtle mental changes such as slight dizziness. Gastrointestinal irritation is a relatively common side effect that may require alteration in therapy.

Corticosteroids given in the small amounts used therapeutically in athletes probably have no effect on performance. Some cyclists competing in multiple-day races have self-injected large doses of corticosteroids in an attempt to decrease their sense of fatigue and soreness. The effects of this practice are unclear and it is considered unethical. (See also Chapter 12.) However, any drug that decreases the athlete's perception of pain has the potential of contributing to chronic injury.

ANTI-MOTION SICKNESS

Many of these drugs cause sedation, which can impair performance. In practice, they can be used at the time of travel as long as competition occurs after the effect of the drug has worn off.

ANTINAUSEANTS

Many are mild sedatives and can impair performance.

ANTIPYRETICS

Aspirin and acetaminophen apparently do not impair performance. However, it is generally felt that an individual with a fever should not exercise.

ANTISPASMODICS AND ANTICHOLINERGICS

The mild sedation associated with many of these drugs suggests that they may impair performance.

ANTITUSSIVES (See under Cough Preparations.)

BETA BLOCKERS (See under Cardiovascular Preparations.)

BRONCHODILATORS (See under Antiasthma.)

CARDIOVASCULAR PREPARATIONS

Beta-adrenergic receptor blocking drugs (beta blockers), such as propranolol, have been used by athletes and musicians to prevent "stage fright" or overstimulation that might interfere with performance requiring fine motor control. Beta blockers diminish the maximal heart rate that an individual can achieve and decrease maximal aerobic capacity. These drugs have been banned by some sports organizations, in particular those involving shooting. (See Chapter 13, which is devoted to cardiovascular preparations.)

COLD PREPARATIONS

Cold medications generally contain an antihistamine and/or decongestant. See under these two headings.

CONTRACEPTIVES, ORAL

The use of these agents has been associated with a lower aerobic capacity[5] and lower static muscle endurance.[6]

CORTICOSTEROID HORMONES (See under Anti-inflammatory Agents.)

COUGH PREPARATIONS

Expectorants increase the flow of bronchial mucus. When used alone, they do not impair performance. However, many cough medications include a cough suppressant that may also act as a sedative. In particular, narcotics used in this way can impair performance.

DECONGESTANTS

Decongestants are sympathomimetic agents that generally have a mild stimulant effect (see Chapter 6). Many are banned at certain international and national competitions.

DERMATOLOGICALS

Most topical drugs are poorly absorbed and do not affect performance.

DIURETICS

The therapeutic use of diuretics does not appear to impair performance. Unfortunately, diuretics sometimes are used to promote dehydration for purposes of extreme weight loss. Dehydration can seriously impair sports performance and may lead to heat injury.[7]

ELECTROLYTES (See Chapter 3.)

GROWTH HORMONE (See Chapter 5.)

HISTAMINE H₂ RECEPTOR ANTAGONISTS

Cimetidine and ranitidine are used in the prevention and treatment of peptic ulcer disease. They are not known to impair athletic performance.

HYPNOTICS

Many sleep medications taken the night before a contest are sufficiently long-acting to impair performance.

IRON PREPARATIONS

These do not impair performance.

MINERALS (See Chapter 3.)

MUSCLE RELAXANTS

These may significantly impair performance owing to general central nervous system depression.

NARCOTICS (See under Analgesics.)

NASAL PREPARATIONS

Most contain decongestants that are sympathomimetic agents. Absorption is small, so there is little systemic stimulation, but they may be detected when drug testing is performed.

OPHTHALMOLOGICALS

These drugs have no effect on performance, but sympathomimetic components may be detected when drug testing is performed.

OTIC PREPARATIONS

These have no effect on performance because they are poorly absorbed.

SEDATIVES

These impair performance owing to central nervous system depression.

STIMULANTS (See Chapter 6.)

SYMPATHOMIMETICS

These are stimulants. Their effects are discussed in Chapter 6. Most are banned at international competitions.

TRANQUILIZERS

These have the potential for impairing sports performance owing to central nervous system depression.

VITAMINS (See Chapter 3.)

REFERENCES

1. Sly RM: Beta-adrenergic drugs in the management of asthma in athletes. J Allergy Clin Immunol 73:680–685, 1984.
2. Kuipers H, Verstappen FTJ, Reneman RS: Influence of therapeutic doses of amoxicillin on aerobic work capacity and some strength characteristics. Am J Sports Med 8:274–279, 1980.
3. Furberg C, Ringqvist T: Penicillin and working capacity. Lancet 1:622, 1967.
4. Sutton JR: Drugs used in metabolic disorders. Med Sci Sports Exerc 13:266–271, 1981.
5. Daggett A, Davies B, Boobis L: Physiological and biochemical responses to exercise following oral contraceptive use. Med Sci Sports Exerc 15:174, 1983.
6. Wirth JC, Lohman TG: The relationship of static muscle function to use of oral contraceptives. Med Sci Sports Exerc 14:16–20, 1982.
7. Caldwell JE, Ahonen E, Nousiainen U: Diuretic therapy, physical performance, and neuromuscular function. Phys Sportsmed 12:73–85, 1984.

12

PHARMACOLOGICAL ADJUNCTS TO THE MANAGEMENT OF MUSCULOSKELETAL INJURIES IN SPORTS

CARL L. STANITSKI, M.D.

I firmly believe that if the whole materia medica, as now used, could be sunk to the bottom of the sea, it would be all the better for mankind—and all the worse for the fishes

OLIVER WENDELL HOLMES—1860.

In pursuit of continued participation in sports, the athlete often joins the legions of Americans who use drugs on a daily basis. Over the past 30 years, there has been a six- to sevenfold increase in drug sales across the United States. Greater than 70 million Americans regularly use over-the-counter and prescription drugs. One of the most commonly taken drugs, aspirin, is the leading over-the-counter cause of adverse drug reactions necessitating hospitalization. It is little wonder that this drug stands out, since 20,000 *tons* of aspirin are ingested annually in the United States.

A marked variability in response to similar drugs by the same patient has been noted. A drug that provides the most relief of symptoms with

173

the best patient tolerance should be selected. Drug side effects such as drowsiness, lethargy, and nausea inhibit an athlete's training and, instead of aiding performance, impair it.

This chapter deals primarily with the effects of inflammation. Classically, these are *calor, tumor, rubor,* and *dolor* (heat, swelling, redness, pain). More specifically, this chapter covers the management of the inflammatory response.

The exact causes of inflammation are multiple and include macro- and microtrauma. These traumatic agents cause loss of continuity of the microvasculature, with leakage of blood elements into interstitial spaces and migration of leukocytes into the tissues. The cycle of swelling, erythema, heat, and pain is then set into motion. Chemical mediators such as histamine, slow-reacting substances, chemotactic factors, kinins, and prostaglandins become locally involved. They cause further leakage of blood elements and fluid, thus promoting the continuing cycle.

Prostaglandins are found in almost every tissue and body fluid. Prostaglandins, fatty acid derivatives of arachidonic acid, in minute amounts produce a wide spectrum of effects in response to a broad range of stimuli. These compounds are autacoids, not hormones, since they are synthesized and exert their actions locally.

Athletes commonly use nonpharmacological modalities to retard or eliminate the inflammatory response. Such methods include ice packs or ice massage, compression wraps, limb elevation, hydrotherapy, contrast baths (alternate heat and cold), and a myriad of immobilization devices.

Since the psyche and body image of the sports participant are often fragile, the placebo effect of any type of treatment, whether pharmacological or not, is often significant. This element must be kept in mind in any assessment of a treatment regimen.

ANALGESICS

It is extremely difficult to quantify pain. A stimulus that is interpreted as mild pain by one person may be considered unbearable by another. As Samuel Johnson noted, "those who do not feel pain seldom think that it is felt."

Analgesics may be divided into two broad categories: mild and strong. Mild analgesics are effective in mild and moderate pain. They decrease the sensitivity of pain receptors through peripheral action and have only minor side effects. Strong analgesics are effective in moderate to severe visceral types of pain by increasing pain tolerance and decreasing anxiety. They also cause changes in consciousness and in apprehension of sensations other than pain because of their central action. Commonly, these drugs must be injected. Strong analgesic medications often produce tolerance and dependence within a week. Dependence may be psychological.

Most of the non-narcotic analgesics (except acetaminophen) also exhibit anti-inflammatory and antipyretic effects. Non-narcotic analgesics are thought to act peripherally, although the brain may be involved as well. Peripheral effects appear to be due to inhibition of prostaglandin synthetase. The prototype of non-narcotic analgesics is acetylsalicylic acid (aspirin). This compound will be discussed further with the anti-inflammatory drugs.

Many analgesics contain mixtures of various compounds, often in arrays that combine short- and long-acting analgesics or other compounds. Such combinations are no more effective than the individual drugs given alone and, in general, should be avoided.

Acetaminophen (Tylenol, Datril) is the active metabolite of phenacetin. Its antipyretic and analgesic activities are equivalent to those of acetylsalicylic acid, but it has weak anti-inflammatory effects. The reason for this is unknown. The side effects of acetaminophen include minor gastrointestinal and allergic responses. Excessive doses of acetaminophen may cause hepatic necrosis and methemoglobinemia. Analgesic nephropathy (renal papillary necrosis and/or interstitial nephritis) occurs with excessive use of acetaminophen or with mixtures of analgesics containing phenacetin, which is metabolized to acetaminophen.

Oxycodone, with or without acetylsalicylic acid (Percodan), phenacetin, or caffeine, is a widely used and abused analgesic that is habituating and addicting. Its use, for other than an extremely short time, should be avoided.

Propoxyphene (Darvon), a methadone congener, has only mild analgesic properties and no anti-inflammatory or antipyretic effects. It is commonly prescribed to bridge the narcotic/non-narcotic gap. Acetylsalicylic acid alone is considered as effective an analgesic as propoxyphene.

SALICYLATES

Naturally occurring acetylsalicylic acid (aspirin) is found in willow bark, which was used to relieve pain and fever over 200 years ago. After the chemical synthesis of aspirin a century ago, it was advocated for the treatment of rheumatic fever. At the beginning of this century, aspirin became a popular substitute for quinine, which had become rare and expensive.

Aspirin should be considered the prime example of the salicylates, all of which produce effects that are analgesic, anti-inflammatory, and antipyretic to varying degrees. The main action of aspirin is to diminish the synthesis or release of prostaglandins and related autacoids. It is bimodal in effect. That is, at low doses it is an effective analgesic, whereas at high doses it is a powerful anti-inflammatory agent.

Plain aspirin dissolves in the stomach and is absorbed in the small intestine. The brand makes little difference. Enteric coating of aspirin delays dissolution until the drug is present in the small bowel and, thus, decreases gastric irritation. However, enteric-coated aspirin requires more time for the analgesic effect to occur and is not satisfactory for single-dose use.

Most buffering agents coupled with aspirin are not present in quantities sufficient to decrease gastric irritation. A full glass of water, milk, or a portion of nonirritating food often is the most effective buffer. When taken 30 to 45 minutes prior to athletic activity, pain and stiffness often can be reduced. Additionally, aspirin at bedtime may help to alleviate the stiffness that occurs the day after vigorous athletic activity.

The most common side effect of aspirin is gastrointestinal irritation, which may progress to include occult blood loss and/or peptic ulcer disease. Gastrointestinal intolerance can be reduced by ingestion of the drug with food, milk, or water. Other side effects include hepatic, hematological, renal, and allergic responses. Transient elevations of liver enzymes return to normal following discontinuation of the drug. Increased serum creatinine and blood urea nitrogen, with diminution of creatinine clearance, may occur with high serum levels of salicylates. Inhibition of platelet aggregation, causing an increase in bleeding time, becomes important in patients pre- and postoperatively. Often, patients forget to divulge chronic aspirin ingestion as part of a routine medical history, since they do not consider aspirin a true drug.

The ready availability of aspirin causes it to be one of the most abused drugs. It accounts for greater than 10,000 cases of intoxication in the United States annually, some severe enough to cause death. Symptoms of mild salicylism include headache, which is paradoxical, since excess ingestion often is related to attempts to eliminate a headache. Other symptoms include nausea, vomiting, tinnitus, and deafness. These effects reverse rapidly when the drug is discontinued.

True salicylate poisoning is associated with vomiting, increased body temperature, excessive sweating, and dehydration. Metabolic acidosis ensues, with increased respiratory rate and compensatory respiratory alkalosis. The cause of death is usually respiratory failure. Treatment involves ventilation, rehydration, and management of the hyperpyrexia. Bicarbonate is given to alkalinize the urine and enhance excretion of the drug.

Diflunisal (Dolobid) is a salicylate that has both anti-inflammatory and analgesic properties. It is probably more effective than simple acetylsalicylic acid for mild to moderate pain, particularly because of its 8- to 12-hour duration of action. It is, however, expensive, and its safety and effectiveness, as compared with other nonsteroidal anti-inflammatory drugs, are unclear.

NONSTEROIDAL ANTI-INFLAMMATORY DRUGS (NSAID's)

Commonly used nonsteroidal anti-inflammatory drugs are listed in Table 12–1. They are bound to plasma protein and inhibit prostaglandin synthesis or release. (Salicylates are NSAID's but are discussed separately, above). The NSAID's have rapid onset of action and also quick dissipation of therapeutic effects once the drug is discontinued. They vary in terms of toxicity, cost, ease of administration, and frequency of

TABLE 12–1. Nonsteroidal Anti-Inflammatory Drugs (NSAID's)

Drug	Trade Name	Supplied as	Suggested Daily Dose	Maximum Daily Dose	Frequency of Administration
Acetylsalicylic acid	Aspirin	325 mg tablet	325–1300 mg	4000 mg*	2–3 tablets q.i.d.*
Diflunisal	Dolobid	250 mg tablet 500 mg tablet	1000 mg	1500 mg	1–2 tablets b.i.d.
Fenoprofen	Nalfon	300 mg capsule 600 mg tablet	2400 mg	3200 mg	2 capsules q.i.d. 1 tablet q.i.d.
Ibuprofen	Motrin	300 mg tablet 400 mg tablet 600 mg tablet	900–1600 mg	2400 mg	1 tablet q.i.d.
Indomethacin	Indocin	25 mg capsule 50 mg capsule	50–100 mg	150 mg	1 capsule b.i.d.
Meclofenamic acid	Meclomen	50 mg capsule 100 mg capsule	200–400 mg	400 mg	1 capsule q.i.d.
Naproxen	Naprosyn	250 mg tablet 500 mg tablet	500 mg	1000 mg	1 tablet b.i.d.
Phenylbutazone	Butazolidin	100 mg tablet	100–400 mg	600 mg	1 tablet q.i.d.
Piroxicam	Feldene	10 mg capsule 20 mg capsule	20 mg	20 mg	20 mg daily in 1–2 doses
Sulindac	Clinoril	150 mg tablet 200 mg tablet	300–400 mg	400 mg	1–2 tablets b.i.d.
Tolmetin	Tolectin	200 mg tablet	1200–1600 mg	2400 mg	2 tablets t.i.d.
	Tolectin DS	400 mg capsule			1 capsule t.i.d.

use. Aspirin should not be used in combination with other NSAID drugs because it reduces serum levels of NSAID's and increases toxicity, including gastrointestinal blood loss. Most of these anti-inflammatory drugs are related to either carboxylic acid or enolic acid (Table 12–2).

NSAID drugs often are compared with aspirin. Aspirin is equally effective in the management of subacute or chronic bursitis and tendinitis from overuse. The NSAID group often is more effective when dealing

TABLE 12–2. NSAID Families

Carboxylic Acids			
SALICYLIC ACIDS AND ESTERS	ACETIC ACIDS	PROPIONIC ACIDS	FENAMIC ACIDS
Aspirin	Alclofenac	Flurbiprofen	Flufenamic
Diflunisal	Diclofenac	Ibuprofen	Meclofenamic
	Fenclofenac	Naproxen	Mefenamic
	Indomethacin		Niflumic
	Sulindac		
	Tolmetin		
Enolic Acids			
PYRAZOLONE	OXICAMS		
Phenylbutazone	Isoxicam		
	Piroxicam		
	Sudoxicam		

with acute bursitis or tendinitis. For full anti-inflammatory activity, 10 or more aspirin tablets may be required per day. Under such circumstances, patient compliance using NSAID's may be better because only 1 to 4 tablets are required per day and gastric irritation may be less. However, the NSAID's are considerably more expensive.

Ibuprofen (Advil) currently is available without prescription after being a prescription-only item (Motrin) for several years. Its popular use for dysmenorrhea has been a factor in its acceptance as a nonprescription item. Current doses are generally tolerated better than salicylates with fewer side effects.

Side effects of the NSAID group occur in about 30 per cent of users. The most common effect is gastrointestinal irritation. Piroxicam, which has a longer half-life, may lead to a higher cumulative dose. Hepatic necrosis, granulomatous chronic hepatitis, and fatal cholestatic jaundice have been reported. Liver enzymes should be monitored during prolonged treatment with these drugs.

NSAID drugs inhibit prostaglandins, which regulate kidney blood flow, glomerular filtration rate, and renal salt and water excretion under conditions of salt and/or volume depletion. Fluid retention, decreased sodium excretion, pre-renal azotemia, hyperkalemia, oliguria, and anuria have been reported with use of these drugs. These effects generally are reversible with discontinuation of the drug and rarely require dialysis. Idiosyncratic nephrotic syndrome or acute interstitial nephritis develops slowly. Occasional cases of acute papillary necrosis have been reported.

Blood dyscrasias are rare but are one of the main causes of death from use of NSAID drugs. All members of this drug family interfere with platelet function and may cause agranulocytosis and aplastic anemia, the latter two usually being on an idiosyncratic basis.

Phenylbutazone (Butazolidine), a second-line anti-inflammatory drug, is commonly cited regarding idiosyncratic agranulocytosis and aplastic anemia. It should be used only over a short period (7 to 10 days), since its desired effects will be noted quickly if the drug is effective. On the other hand, piroxicam may require a one-week period to provide levels high enough to achieve its anti-inflammatory effect.

Other side effects of NSAID drugs include dermatitis, headaches, tinnitus, and lightheadedness. Allergic reaction with bronchospasm may occur in patients with such responses to aspirin. In general, the nonsteroidal anti-inflammatory drugs are usually well tolerated. In patients undergoing treatment with such drugs, periodic white blood cell counts, serum creatinine, and liver enzyme tests should be done to detect toxic effects.

Relative contraindications to the use of nonsteroidal anti-inflammatory drugs include childhood, pregnancy, pre-existing renal or hepatic pathology, and active peptic ulcer disease.

CORTICOSTEROIDS

More than 25 years ago, Hench and coworkers, in Nobel Prize winning work at the Mayo Clinic, demonstrated the beneficial effects of cortisone and ACTH on rheumatoid arthritis. They found that these corticosteroid hormones inhibited phospholipase and blocked synthesis of prostaglandins. After an initial burst of enthusiasm for the systemic and regional use of corticosteroids, complications were noted. Adverse effects included the production of fulminant infections, severe osteoporosis, proximal myopathy, glucose intolerance, hypertension, capillary fragility, psychological changes, hirsutism, cataracts, pancreatitis, growth inhibition, diminished wound healing, and withdrawal phenomena. Such effects were dose-related in systemically administered drugs.

Deleterious effects of intra-articular, peritendon, and intratendon injections were seen. Intra-articular use stabilized the synovial membrane and prevented acid hydrolase release. However, cartilage matrix production and organization were inhibited owing to the steroid effect on chondrocyte metabolism. In addition, intra-articular injections may provide an analgesic effect and mask the protective pain associated with injury. Such unwarranted analgesia encourages the athlete to continue participation, with acceleration of the degeneration produced by the initial injury. The "shooting up" of athletes in the 1950's and 1960's was not intravenously, as noted in the recreational drug culture, but rather was intra-articular, which allowed the athlete to attempt to return to play. This practice is to be soundly condemned, and it is hoped the practice is a rare occurrence today.

The pain commonly noted following an intra-articular injection seems to be related to phagocytosis of the injected crystals by polymorphonuclear neutrophils. Such pain is usually managed with ice and salicylates.

The use of corticosteroids for treating soft-tissue injuries must be judicious. Corticosteroids inhibit collagen formation in granulation tissue and retard wound healing. In addition, wound healing requires an orderly inflammatory response with secondary controlled "inflammation." The use of corticosteroids interferes with this orderly process and is detrimental to wound healing.

Many acute tendon ruptures have followed the injection of steroids into tendons of upper or lower extremities. Such injections markedly change the biomechanical properties of the tendons and render them susceptible to rupture. Because of the analgesic effect of the corticosteroid, unwarranted return to play may occur with further stress applied to a compromised tendon. When dealing with severe tendinitis, peritendinous—and not intratendinous—injections should be done as a last resort. Following the injection, the athlete must be advised against vigorous activity for the next two to three weeks to allow resolution of the inflammatory state of the tendon so that potential disruption of the tendon does not occur.

Noyes et al. in animal studies with high doses of corticosteroids noted significant diminution of mechanical properties in anterior cruciate ligaments. When a dosage was used equivalent to that employed in treatment of human joints, biomechanical changes were present but did not significantly compromise the bone-ligament-bone unit.

Since corticosteroids are lipolytic, subcutaneous loss of fat and depigmentation may occur, particularly about the lateral epicondyle of the elbow. Steroid injections into the calcaneal fat pad cause dissolution of the fat cushion and actually aggravate calcaneal bursitis because of loss of the heel pad's dampening effect.

Repeated injections near the lateral epicondyle of the elbow may lead to spontaneous rupture of the wrist extensor mechanism, particularly in patients who persist in playing racquet sports during the course of treatment.

Corticosteroid injection is contraindicated when skin infection is present at the injection site. The possibility of a septic joint must be ruled out prior to any intra-articular steroid injection. Painful joint effusion and fever following injection suggest joint infection.

With the advent of nonsteroidal anti-inflammatory drugs, the need for systemic corticosteroid administration to manage musculoskeletal problems has diminished markedly. In only rare instances is a short course of oral steroids required. If this is necessary, a high loading dose should be given over the first several days, followed by rapid tapering over the next week to 10 days.

In patients who have taken an oral corticosteroid for a prolonged period of time, suppression of the pituitary-adrenal axis is present, and withdrawal of the steroid should be done gradually. In such patients, a preoperative steroid "boost" is required. Tapering of the steroid dose should be done postoperatively to prevent withdrawal symptoms and potential adrenal collapse.

DIMETHYL SULFOXIDE (DMSO)

The ability to penetrate intact skin is a unique property of dimethyl sulfoxide. Over the past 20 years, DMSO has been claimed variously to be a wonder drug or a hoax. Early clinical trials in 1964 and 1965 on more than 100,000 patients with a variety of conditions were undertaken. Studies were discontinued when a change in the refractive index of the lenses of laboratory animals treated with DMSO was noted. No similar changes had been noted in humans.

In 1980, the U.S. Food and Drug Administration approved the use of a 50 per cent solution of DMSO for irrigation in interstitial cystitis. In Canada, DMSO is approved as a 70 per cent cutaneous solution for scleroderma. A 90 per cent DMSO gel for topical application is utilized by veterinarians to reduce local swelling secondary to trauma.

The DMSO preparation most commonly sold and used by the public is a 99 per cent industrial strength solution used for degreasing. No guarantee of this compound's purity is made. Because of DMSO's trans-cutaneous migration, contaminants also may be absorbed.

Adverse responses include a garlic odor and taste in the mouth. Localized skin irritation also occurs because of the drying and degreasing actions of the solvent.

Currently, centers are involved in prospective, well-controlled studies of the effect of DMSO on head injuries and on cutaneous ulcers in scleroderma. Studies are also expected on the effect of DMSO in chronic and acute musculoskeletal injuries and disorders.

The safety and efficacy of DMSO for musculoskeletal problems have not been established. Until the controversy is resolved, it would seem prudent to avoid use of this compound.

SKELETAL MUSCLE RELAXANTS

The use of this group of compounds to treat painful muscle contractions due to local inflammatory responses, as commonly encountered in athletic injuries, is controversial. Most muscle relaxants are neuronal depressants that act centrally and interfere with reflexes. Drugs to manage spasticity of central origin are not indicated for the treatment of local skeletal muscle spasm.

Muscle spasm secondary to trauma or its inflammatory response is thought to be due to local involuntary contraction and is not accompanied by signs of spasticity, such as increased stretch reflex. Since such spasms are often of brief duration and self-limited, it is difficult to assess the clinical response to a drug alone.

Chlordiazepoxide (Limbitrol), chlorzoxazone with acetaminophen (Parafon), methocarbamol (Robaxin), and orphenadrine citrate (Disipal) with aspirin, phenacetin, and caffeine have no greater efficacy than simple aspirin or placebo. Carisoprodol (Soma) with aspirin has a central action and has not been demonstrated to directly relax localized tense skeletal muscles in man. The relief of muscle spasm may be secondary to a central sedative effect or to the anti-inflammatory effect of the associated salicylate. Cyclobenzaprine (Flexeril) is closely related to the tricyclic antidepressants and, in addition to the similar side effects of those compounds, causes sedation. There are no data to demonstrate its effectiveness in isolated skeletal muscle spasms.

The effectiveness of diazepam (Valium) has not been assessed for long-term use (greater than four months). This benzodiazepine derivative has side effects similar to those noted with barbiturates, that is, ataxia, drowsiness, fatigue, and headaches. It potentiates central nervous system depressants, including alcohol. The action of diazepam is potentiated by barbiturates, MAO inhibitors, phenothiazines, and narcotics.

Since rest, analgesics, spontaneous improvement of the local skeletal spasm, and drug-placebo effects are often all involved, it is difficult to ascertain the value of muscle relaxants in the management of athletic injuries. Because of significant associated central nervous system side effects such as drowsiness, which may prove dangerous, the role for this family of drugs in the management of athletic injuries seems quite limited.

Aspirin, because of its zone of safety, inexpensiveness, and effectiveness, remains the drug of choice for the management of routine musculoskeletal pain and inflammation. Nonsteroidal anti-inflammatory drugs and corticosteroids occasionally may be necessary, but their efficacy must be judged against the standard of aspirin.

FURTHER READINGS

Acetylsalicylic acid. Medical Letter 23, 15:65066, July 24, 1981.

Cox JS: Current concepts in the role of steroids in the treatment of sprains and strains. Med Sci Sports Exerc 16(3):216–218, June 1984.

Drug Facts and Comparisons. Philadelphia, Lippincott, 1984.

Flexeril (Cyclobenzaprine). Medical Letter 20, 3:12, February 3, 1978.

Ismail AM, Balakrishnan R, Rajakumar MK: Rupture of patellar ligament after steroid infiltration. J Bone Joint Surg 51B:503–505, 1969.

Kapetanos G: The effect of the local corticosteroids on the healing and biomechanical properties of the partially injured tendon. Clin Orthop 163(3):170–179, 1982.

Lasagna L: Controversies in Therapeutics. Philadelphia, W. B. Saunders Company, 1980.

Mankin HJ, Conger KA: The acute effects of intraarticular hydrocortisone on articular cartilage in rabbits. J Bone Joint Surg 48A:1383–1388, 1966.

Miller R, Greenblatt DJ: Handbook of Drug Therapy. New York, Elsevier, 1979.

Noyes FR, Grouw ES, Nussbaum NS, Cooper SM: Effect of intra-articular corticosteroids on ligament properties. Clin Orthop 123:197–209, 1977.

Salter RB, Gross A, Hall JH: Hydrocortisone arthropathy—an experimental investigation. Can Med Assoc J 97:374, 1967.

13

DRUGS, EXERCISE, AND THE CARDIOVASCULAR SYSTEM

DAVID T. LOWENTHAL, M.D. Ph.D.
JONATHAN PARMET, M.D.
ESTHER PARAN, M.D.
ZEBULON KENDRICK, PH.D.

This chapter covers the effects of cardiovascular drugs on exercise, stress testing, and physical training, particularly in persons with cardiovascular disease. Responses to nontherapeutic drugs such as caffeine, nicotine, alcohol, and marijuana also are discussed.

In patients with cardiovascular diseases such as hypertension or those undergoing cardiac rehabilitation, it is beneficial to allow activity without the adverse effects of extreme increases in pulse rate, blood pressure, catecholamines, and potassium. As a result, drugs are sought that allow the patient to exercise while keeping the increase in exercise-induced parameters modest, protecting an often-times compromised and vulnerable myocardium.

In general, all of the drugs consumed by patients with cardiovascular disease, with the exception of beta-adrenergic blocking agents, permit a normal exercise response. The normal acute response is an increase in systolic blood pressure with little or no fall in diastolic pressure and an increase in heart rate, stroke index, and cardiac index. Following a conditioning program, appropriate changes occur during physical activity but are less pronounced for a given level of exercise.

Most studies have investigated the effects of drugs during acute episodes of exercise. The literature also contains a few short-term chronic studies. A training effect from dynamic physical activity is possible when the patient is on a beta-adrenergic blocking agent such as propranolol (Inderal) or atenolol (Tenormin). Even when antihypertensives, calcium-channel blocking drugs, digitalis preparations, antiarrhythmic agents, or nitrates are prescribed, usually there is no embarrassment to the acute response during stress testing, although training effects may be blunted.

EFFECTS OF CARDIOVASCULAR DRUGS ON EXERCISE

DIURETICS

Diuretics are widely used antihypertensives. Their actions during exercise may vary.[1] Thiazides cause a drop in exercise blood pressure by decreasing peripheral resistance and plasma volume. Long-term use of thiazides does not cause a drop in cardiac output. The effects of furosemide (Lasix) on exercise have not been well studied.

With any diuretic therapy, hypokalemia can become significant, resulting in moderate ST segment depression, cardiac irritability, and skeletal muscle fatigue. During vigorous exercise, serum potassium increases. The source is skeletal muscle. This can occur in the presence of diuretic-induced hypokalemia, indicating that total-body potassium is not depleted.[2] However, to ensure against potassium loss, patients on diuretics should receive potassium supplements.

Thus, diuretics result in a moderate decrease in the blood pressure response to exercise and, with adequate potassium supplementation, should not provoke any drug-related risks during physical activity.

CENTRAL ALPHA-AGONISTS

Many studies dealing with the central alpha-agonist antihypertensive drugs have been performed recently. Guanabenz (Wytensin), clonidine (Catapres), and alpha-methyldopa (methyldopa, Aldomet) decrease central and/or peripheral outflow of catecholamines. This results in reductions of plasma norepinephrine at rest and during exercise.[3,4] All of these drugs can blunt the sympathetic response during exercise, but they have significantly different hemodynamic effects.

In mild hypertensives, methyldopa may decrease the blood pressure and heart rate response to exercise.[5] Total peripheral resistance and cardiac output may[6] or may not[7] decrease. Clonidine differs from methyldopa in that it reduces blood pressure and heart rate at rest as well as during exercise.[8,9] Central vagal stimulation results in decreased heart rate and a drop in cardiac output.[10] However, this is not considered a negative inotropic property, since cardiac output is normalized after chronic use. In contrast to clonidine, guanabenz does not decrease heart rate or cardiac output at rest or during dynamic exercise.

Clonidine and methyldopa did not affect the changes in serum potassium, renin, and aldosterone that are normally observed in healthy persons.[4,9,11] No significant ST-T changes occurred during exercise using these drugs. The rise in diastolic blood pressure induced by isometric activity may be decreased with clonidine or methyldopa.

BETA BLOCKERS

The most important effect of beta-adrenergic blocking drugs is that cardiac output is reduced during exercise without any peripheral vascular effects. The basis for this is that myocardial contractility and heart rate are reduced. Both of these changes cause a longer diastolic phase, which allows better coronary perfusion. This is an advantage for patients with coronary artery disease who are undergoing cardiac rehabilitation. With beta blockade, many such patients can exercise longer, have less angina, and have fewer incidents of ST depression.[12] In patients with ischemic heart disease on propranolol, physical training can result in up to a 31 per cent improvement in exercise capacity.[13] Even the elderly and patients with atrial fibrillation can achieve a significant training effect.[14]

Propranolol and the cardioselective beta blockers atenolol and metoprolol (Lopressor) have been studied in normal volunteers. Heart rate and systolic blood pressure were reduced at maximum exercise.[4,15] There were no significant changes in diastolic blood pressure, oxygen consumption, or anaerobic threshold (that point at which oxygen consumption fails to increase in proportion to minute ventilation).[4,15] This indicates that blood flow to the active muscles was unaltered.

There is marked individual variability of beta-blocking effects on heart rate and blood pressure during exercise.[16] Cardioselective beta blockers appear to be more effective than nonselective agents in blunting the increase in systolic blood pressure.

Isometric exercise, such as trying to lift a heavy load that will not move, is known to increase blood pressure. Antihypertensive therapy may decrease this response in persons with cardiovascular disease.[3,17] However, in patients with borderline hypertensive heart failure, metoprolol, with or without prazosin (Minipress) vasodilatory treatment, did not safely abolish dangerous increases in blood pressure during isometric activity.[18–21]

Metabolic effects of beta blockade during exercise include the following: Propranolol may increase serum potassium more than dynamic exercise does alone. Renin is decreased,[4] although plasma aldosterone does not appear to change. In contrast to the central alpha agonists, propranolol and metoprolol either increase plasma norepinephrine[22] or permit normal increases in plasma values[4,23] during physical activity.

Although beta blockade increases endurance in cardiac patients, it causes exercise fatigue in normal individuals. This appears to be due to substrate limitation—decreased blood levels of glucose, nonesterified fatty acids, and glycerol. Muscle glycogenolysis, a $beta_2$-adrenoreceptor–mediated process, probably also decreases.

Neither propranolol nor metoprolol decreases the ventilatory response to CO_2 during physical activity.[24] This may be significant in the management of patients with chronic obstructive pulmonary disease in whom these drugs will not worsen CO_2 retention. In normal volunteers, a single dose of propranolol reduced oxygen consumption at both submaximal and maximal efforts.[25]

Plasma levels of both propranolol and acebutolol increase during exercise. This may be related to pH changes or to decreased hepatic blood flow during activity, which would affect those drugs with a high hepatic extraction ratio.

VASODILATORS

The vasodilators are used adjunctively with other drugs in the treatment of hypertension and include hydralazine (Apresoline), minoxidil (Loniten), and prazosin. In normal volunteers, hydralazine decreases arterial pressure, with a resultant reflex tachycardia. This tends to increase cardiac output through an increase in sympathetic drive, which, in a compromised heart, may lead to myocardial ischemia with angina and/or infarction.[26] However, the drug is useful as an afterload reducer in chronic heart failure.[27]

Prazosin is more of an atypical alpha-antagonist than a direct-acting vasodilator. It decreases mean arterial blood pressure and total peripheral resistance at rest and with dynamic work.[28] In contrast to hydralazine, there is no reflex increase in heart rate or pressor response greater than with a placebo.[29] During isometric activity, hydralazine neither improves skeletal muscle oxygen delivery in patients with heart failure[30] nor adequately attenuates increases in sympathetic activity.[18,31]

In heart failure patients, vasodilators are of interest during exercise. While increasing cardiac output by reducing afterload, hydralazine reduces both arterial and pulmonary wedge pressure and increases stroke volume.[27] However, exercise tolerance appears not to improve. Its vasodilatory effect does not add to that of local metabolites.[30]

In patients with borderline hypertensive heart failure, prazosin improves cardiac output and moderates the increase in diastolic blood pressure associated with isometric activity. Minoxidil, a most potent direct vasodilator, may improve exercise tolerance in patients with chronic heart failure owing to its afterload-reducing properties.

ANGIOTENSIN-CONVERTING-ENZYME INHIBITORS

Captopril (Capoten) is an angiotensin-converting-enzyme inhibitor. Investigators disagree on its effects on dynamic exercise. Several studies indicate a reduction in systolic and diastolic blood pressure during exercise.[32, 33] Similar decreases in blood pressure with dynamic activity were seen with saralasin, an angiotensin II partial antagonist.[34] The reduction in angiotensin II with captopril and saralasin, with an unaltered blood pressure response to exercise, indicates that angiotensin II is not a major determinant of blood pressure regulation during exercise in hypertensive patients. Captopril also was found to reduce plasma aldosterone levels at rest and during physical activity.[32] Plasma renin activity increased, while concentrations of norepinephrine and epinephrine remained unchanged. Similar responses have been seen with enalapril (Vasotec).

Calcium Antagonists

The calcium antagonists verapamil (Calan, Isoptin) and nifedipine (Procardia) have differing clinical applications. Verapamil is an antiarrhythmic agent that is particularly useful in paroxysmal atrial tachycardia. Both verapamil and nifedipine are used in the management of angina, myocardial infarction, and coronary artery bypass graft surgery to prevent further ischemia and to augment collateral myocardial blood flow.[35] Their effects are important in the rehabilitation of cardiac patients. In normal, active persons, both verapamil and nifedipine have little effect on blood pressure at rest or during exercise.[36] Both drugs help to alleviate chronic angina[37, 38] by decreasing afterload and reducing myocardial oxygen demand. Exercise-induced angina and ST depression are diminished.[38, 39] Left ventricular diastolic filling may be enhanced. Serum potassium levels are similar to those with placebo. Thus, verapamil and nifedipine may be used during training programs with cardiac patients without risk of dangerous increases in blood pressure or serum potassium as compared to placebo.

Nitrates

The nitrates are represented by nitroglycerine and isosorbide dinitrate (Isordil, Sorbide, Sorbitrate). In normal humans, their hemodynamic effects are attributable largely to their venodilatory actions. Effects include reduced mean arterial pressure, decreased cardiac filling, and increased heart rate.[40] During dynamic activity, cardiac output is unchanged because these parameters balance out.[41]

More important, however, are the effects of nitrates in patients with coronary artery disease and/or heart failure. Nitroglycerine is effective in controlling angina pectoris, and, consequently, it also increases exercise duration when chest pain is the limiting factor. These actions are thought to result from a decrease in preload which gives rise to a reduction in left ventricular end-diastolic pressure.[41]

Isosorbide dinitrate is a long-acting nitrate with similar effects on exercise. In patients with congestive heart failure, changes are not seen during initial treatment. However, after three months of treatment, cardiac output, oxygen consumption, and exercise duration improve.[42]

In patients with angina due to coronary heart disease, an individual dose of isosorbide dinitrate significantly improved exercise tolerance. It also reduced resting systolic pressure and increased heart rate. In exercising patients, nitrates will not worsen ST segment changes. In fact, ECG evidence of myocardial ischemia following exercise is reduced in patients with angina who received large doses of isosorbide dinitrate.[43]

Digitalis

In normal individuals, digitalis reduces heart rate and cardiac output without changing blood pressure.[44] It also produces ST segment depression during exercise in persons with normal coronary vessels.[12]

In patients with congestive heart failure, digitalization reduces ventricle size and oxygen consumption at baseline[45] and decreases left ventricular end-diastolic pressure during exercise.[46] Unfortunately, no changes in exercise tolerance have been noted in these patients.[47] Arrhythmias associated with the drug can be provoked by exercise, especially with concurrent diuretic-induced potassium depletion.[48] Therefore, patients who take digitalis should be monitored carefully in any training program with regard to electrolyte values and for ectopy.

ANTIARRHYTHMICS

Procainamide (Pronestyl) and quinidine cause no change in heart rate or oxygen uptake during dynamic exercise, but systolic blood pressure may drop slightly.[49, 50] Exercise-induced arrhythmias decrease in number and severity. Thus, in patients with demonstrable ectopy not corrected by overdrive suppression, these drugs may be used effectively to reduce the risk of exercise-induced arrhythmias. Both procainamide and quinidine can mask exercise-induced ST segment depression, producing a false-negative stress test.[51, 52]

CONCLUSION

The graded treadmill or cycle ergometry exercise test must be interpreted in the context of the drug regimen the patient is following. An appreciation of the hemodynamic and/or biochemical changes induced by drugs is critical for a logical critique of the performance of the patient and for the projected exercise prescription. Drug therapy clearly is not a contraindication to acute or chronic exercise as long as the principles of basic exercise physiology in unmedicated persons can be translated to the medicated patient.

ERGOGENIC (PERFORMANCE) AIDS THAT AFFECT THE CARDIOVASCULAR SYSTEM

The consumption of drugs by participants in sports is rampant, despite physicians' efforts to provide rational therapy and despite warnings. In the remainder of this chapter, drugs that alter performance are discussed, with particular reference to the cardiovascular system.

CAFFEINE

Caffeine has long been considered an ergogenic (energy) aid or doping agent[53] that could enhance athletic performance.[54-57] However, the ergogenic effects of caffeine and related methylxanthines are unclear. The lack of clarity may be due to caffeine-induced physiological responses that are influenced by dose,[58, 59] differ from habitual to nonhabitual users,[59-63] and elicit both direct and indirect effects. The significant effects of caffeine on the cardiovascular system are summarized in Table 13–1.

TABLE 13–1. Caffeine and the Cardiovascular System

Effects of Caffeine on the Peripheral Vascular System

Decreases peripheral vascular resistance
Increases perfusion to most organs
Increases cerebrovascular resistance
No change in blood pressure with habitual use

Effects of Caffeine on Cardiac Function (Habitual Use)

Increases heart rate
Arrhythmogenic
Increases coronary blood flow (possibly from increased work and vascular smooth
    muscle relaxation)
Increases isovolumetric contraction
Increases contractile force (possibly related to catecholamines)

ALCOHOL

Alcohol is a myocardial depressant. The impaired myocardial performance includes a decrease in stroke work with concomitant increase in left ventricular end-diastolic pressure and a decrease in left ventricular work and tension-time index.[64–66] Alcohol consumption also increases skin blood flow and sweating.[67, 68] Heart rate and cardiac output are higher at rest and during submaximal exercise. Total arteriovenous oxygen difference and total peripheral resistance decrease. During maximal work, pulmonary ventilation is reduced, but circulatory responses are not affected.[69,70]

When used chronically, alcohol can act as a vasoconstrictor and produce hypertension. The elevated blood pressure is reversible upon cessation of alcohol consumption.

AMPHETAMINES AND RELATED STIMULANTS

Amphetamines and related stimulants may be consumed in large quantities by some athletes, but their effects are controversial and dangerous.[71, 72] Amphetamines originally were used for weight control, but they are no longer recommended for this purpose. They are useful in the treatment of narcolepsy and hyperactivity in children. The customary dose of Benzedrine or Dexedrine is 15 mg, but professional football players have been alleged to consume 150 mg of amphetamines per game.[73] The short-term effects of an average 15-mg dose (Table 13–2) include decreased appetite, increased alertness and confidence, elevated mood, improved physical performance and concentration, and decreased

TABLE 13–2. Amphetamines: Short-term Effects of an Average Dose (15 mg)

Anorexia
Increase in alertness and confidence
Improved physical performance (certain types) and concentration
Decreased sense of fatigue
Feeling of anxiousness

TABLE 13–3. Amphetamines: Short-term Effects of a Large Dose (150 mg)

Acute paranoia, agitation, fear
Irritability
Acute hypertension
Fever, chills, headache
Chest pain
Death (rarely)

sense of fatigue. Yet associated with these effects is the feeling of anxiousness or of generally being on "a high."

The short-term effects of large amounts (150 mg) of amphetamines (Table 13–3) include profound overstimulation, acute paranoia, agitation, insomnia, fear, and irritability. Also, there is a sharp rise in blood pressure, fever, chest pain, headache, chills, and stomach distress. Rhabdomyolysis may occur as a result of the direct toxic effect of the amphetamine on skeletal muscle. Rarely, death occurs.

With long-term abuse of amphetamines, tolerance develops. Psychological dependence on, and preoccupation with, these drugs is customary. The user may suffer from paranoia, auditory and visual hallucinations, and formication. The withdrawal syndrome is well known. It would be senseless to belabor the point that amphetamines are deleterious to the athlete as well as to the nonathlete when improperly consumed.

Cocaine has effects similar to those of the amphetamines, but the subjective manifestations are more intense. This may be due to the way in which cocaine is taken—through the nasal mucosa or lungs. The onset of action is more rapid and the duration of effect is shorter for the average dose.

Short-term effects of large amounts of cocaine are similar to those of the amphetamines. However, an initial tachycardia may be replaced by a slow, weak heart beat, and respiration may change from an initial tachypnea to shallow, slow breathing.

NICOTINE

Epidemiological studies in the last 10 years demonstrate that cigarette smoking is a substantial risk factor for atherogenesis, acute ischemic heart disease, and sudden cardiac death.[74, 75] It is postulated that smoking contributes to acute events through thrombotic occlusion of coronary arteries, myocardial oxygen depletion, and an enhanced tendency for ventricular arrhythmias.[76] The risk of coronary heart disease is increased by other risk factors and decreased by the cessation of smoking.

The two major toxic constituents of cigarette smoke are carbon monoxide and nicotine.[77] Intake of carbon monoxide elevates carboxyhemoglobin levels, which interfere with myocardial oxygen supply, especially in the presence of partially occluded coronary arteries. This effect of carbon monoxide is additive to the cardiovascular actions of nicotine, which increase myocardial oxygen demand through sympathetic and parasympathetic stimulation of the heart. The smoking of one or two cigarettes or the administration of an equivalent amount of nicotine by other means causes significant sympathomimetic symptoms: increase of resting heart rate from 5 to 40 beats per minute; increase in blood pressure of 5 to 20 mm Hg; and increased serum levels of norepinephrine and epinephrine, causing significant vasoconstriction. The combination of mild stress and cigarette smoking produces marked hemodynamic effects larger than either factor alone.[74] This synergistic effect probably is due to their similar actions on the sympathetic nervous system.[76]

In addition to its peripheral action, nicotine has a direct effect on the central nervous system. Nicotine from smoking produces central nervous system arousal, expressed on EEG as desynchronization of cortical electric activity and as release of the neuropeptides vasopressin and beta-endorphin. Yet rather than producing expected increases of emotional behavior and feelings, most smokers report that they smoke to reduce negative affect or to achieve pleasurable relaxation.[78] Less than 25 per cent of smokers report stimulation from cigarette smoking. Animal studies have shown that nicotine reduces aggression and indices of fear and anxiety without changing general activity levels. The paradoxical tranquilizing effect of nicotine is not understood.

CANNABIS (MARIJUANA)

The use of marijuana in herbal medicine is long-standing. For centuries it was used in Asia, the Near East, and Africa, and it was imported to Europe in the early 1800's. During the nineteenth century, marijuana was used widely in western medicine as an analgesic, anti-convulsant, sedative hypnotic, topical analgesic, and bronchodilator. In the 1930's, it was supposed that recreational use of marijuana led to the abuse of narcotics. Its use was declared illegal for any purpose. However, according to nationwide surveys conducted in the early 1970's, 23 per cent of youth and 53 per cent of young adults had tried marijuana at least once. About 10 per cent of these groups considered themselves regular users.[79]

After a marijuana cigarette is smoked, there is a sharp elevation in the blood level of delta-tetrahydrocannabinol, the major psychoactive ingredient of marijuana. It disappears from the circulation within two to three hours, the time frame that coincides with behavioral effects. Smoking marijuana changes various body system activities. Some of these changes have been studied thoroughly, whereas others still are controversial.

CARDIOVASCULAR EFFECTS OF MARIJUANA

The typical effect of marijuana in humans is tachycardia.[80] Some investigators reported ECG changes, including T-wave and ST-segment alterations and premature ventricular contractions. Owing to the tachycardia there is an increase in left ventricular ejection time and cardiac output by 28 and 30 per cent, respectively. Since the marijuana-induced tachycardia cannot be blocked by propranolol, its mechanism must be other than beta-adrenergic stimulation. However, plasma norepinephrine concentrations are increased with marijuana.

Peak exercise performance is decreased by marijuana because premature achievement of maximum heart rate during exercise diminishes maximum exercise capacity. Patients with angina pectoris develop symptoms at lower exercise levels after smoking marijuana, indicating increased myocardial oxygen consumption due to the drug. Marijuana can produce postural hypotension when given in large doses and can inhibit the normal vasoconstrictor response to ice water as well.

CONCLUSION

We have attempted to review significant developments in the burgeoning field of exercise pharmacology. In particular, cardiovascular pharmacology and ergogenic aids to performance are discussed.

REFERENCES

1. Lund-Johansen P: Hemodynamic changes in long-term diuretic therapy of essential hypertension. A comparative study of chlorthalidone, polythiazide and hydrochlorothiazide. Acta Med Scand 187:509–518, 1970.
2. Falkner B, Onesti G, Lowenthal DT, Affrime MB: Effectiveness of centrally acting drugs and diuretics in adolescent hypertension. Clin Pharmacol Ther 32:577–583, 1982.
3. Virtanen K, Janne J, Frick MH: Response of blood pressure and plasma norepinephrine to propranolol, metoprolol and clonidine during isometric and dynamic exercise. Eur J Clin Pharmacol 21:275–279, 1982.
4. Lowenthal DT, Affrime MB, Falkner B, Saris S, Hakki H, et al: Potassium disposition and neuroendocrine effects of propranolol, methyldopa and clonidine during dynamic exercise. Clin Exp Hypertens Theor Pract A4(9&10):1895–1911, 1982.
5. Sannerstedt R, Varnanskes E, Werko L: Hemodynamic effects of methyldopa (Aldomet) at rest and during exercise in patients with arterial hypertension. Acta Med Scand 171:75–82, 1962.
6. Lund-Johansen P: Hemodynamic changes in long-term alpha methyldopa therapy of essential hypertension. Acta Med Scand 192:221–226, 1972.
7. Chamberlain DA, Howard J: Guanethidine and methyldopa: A haemodynamic study. Br Heart J 26:528–536, 1964.
8. Lund-Johansen P: Hemodynamic changes at rest and during exercise in long-term clonidine therapy of essential hypertension. Acta Med Scand 195:111–117, 1974.
9. Lowenthal DT, Affrime MB, Rosenthal L, Gould AB, Borruso J, et al: Dynamic and biochemical responses to single and repeated doses of clonidine during dynamic physical activity. Clin Pharmacol Ther 32:18–24, 1982.
10. Onesti G, Schwartz AB, Kim KE, Paz-Martinez V, Swarz C: Antihypertensive effect of clonidine. Circ Res 28 (Suppl 2):53–69, 1971.
11. Rosenthal L, Affrime MB, Lowenthal DT, Falkner B, Saris S., et al: Biochemical and dynamic responses to single and repeated doses of methyldopa and propranolol during dynamic physical activity. Clin Pharmacol Ther 32:701–710, 1982.
12. Ellestad MH (ed): Stress Testing. Principles and Practice, 2nd ed. Philadelphia, F.A. Davis Company, 1980.
13. Pratt CM, Welton DE, Squires WG Jr, Kirby TE, Hartung GH, et al: Demonstration of training effect during chronic beta-adrenergic blockade in patients with coronary artery disease. Circulation 64:1125–1129, 1981.

14. Hare TW, Lowenthal DT, Hakki HH, Goodwin M: Demonstration of training effect in elderly patients with coronary artery disease receiving beta adrenergic blocking drugs. Ann Sports Med 2(1):36–40, 1984.
15. Sklar J, Johnston DG, Overlie P, Gerber JG, Brammell HL, et al: The effects of a cardioselective (metoprolol) and a nonselective (propranolol) beta-adrenergic blocker on the response to dynamic exercise in normal men. Circulation 65:894–899, 1982.
16. Kramer B, Kramer G, Walz G, Stankov G, Welsch M, et al: Analysis of inter-individual variability of beta blocking effects on heart rate and blood pressure during exercise (Abstract). J Am Col Cardiol 1:625, 1983.
17. Lowenthal DT, Saris SD, Packer J, Haratz A, Conry K: The mechanisms of action and the clinical pharmacology of beta adrenergic blocking drugs. Am J Med 77(4A):119–127, 1984.
18. O'Hare JA, Murnaghan DJ: Failure of antihypertensive drugs to control blood pressure rise with isometric exercise in hypertension. Postgrad Med J 57:552–555, 1981.
19. Nelson GIC, Donnelly GL, Hunyor SN: Haemodynamic effects of sustained treatment with prazosin and metoprolol, alone and in combination, in borderline hypertensive heart failure. J Cardiovasc Pharmacol 4:240–245, 1982.
20. Hansson BG, Dymling JF, Manhem P, Hokfelt B: Long-term treatment of moderate hypertension with the beta$_1$-receptor blocking agent metoprolol. II. Effect of submaximal work and insulin-induced hypoglycaemia on plasma catecholamines and renin activity, blood pressure and pulse rate. Eur J Clin Pharmacol 11:247–254, 1977.
21. Lijnen PG, Amery AK, Fagard RH, Reybrouck TM, Moerman EF, et al: The effect of beta-adrenoceptor blockade on renin, angiotensin, aldosterone and catecholamines at rest and during exercise. Br J Clin Pharmacol 7:175–181, 1979.
22. Christensen NJ, Brandsborg O: The relationship between plasma catecholamine concentration and pulse rate during exercise and standing. Eur J Clin Invest 3:299–306, 1973.
23. Lundborg P, Astrom H, Bengtsson C, Fellenius E, Von Schenck H, et al: Effect of beta-adrenoceptor blockade on exercise performance and metabolism. Clin Sci 61:299–305, 1981.
24. Leitch AG, Hopkin JM, Ellis DA, Clarkson D McG, Merchant S, et al: Failure of propranolol and metoprolol to alter ventilatory responses to carbon dioxide and exercise. Br J Clin Pharmacol 9:493–498, 1980.
25. Twentyman OP, Disley A, Gribbin HR, Alberti KMGG: Effect of beta adrenergic blockade on respiratory and metabolic responses to exercise. J Appl Physiol 51:788–793, 1981.
26. Moyer JH: Hydralazine (Apresoline) hydrochloride. Pharmacological observations and clinical results in the therapy of hypertension. Arch Intern Med 91:419–439, 1953.
27. Ginks WR, Redwood DR: Haemodynamic effects of hydralazine at rest and during exercise in patients with chronic heart failure. Br Heart J 44:259–264, 1980.
28. Lund-Johansen P: Hemodynamic changes at rest and during exercise in long-term prazosin therapy for essential hypertension. Postgraduate Medicine Symposium on Prazosin, November, 1975, p 45.
29. Lowenthal DT: Hypertension and Exercise. In Bove AA, Lowenthal DT (eds): Exercise Medicine: Physiologic Principles and Clinical Applications. New York, Academic Press, 1984.
30. Wilson JR, Untereker W, Hurshfeld J: Effects of isosorbide dinitrate and hydralazine on regional metabolic responses to arm exercise in patients with heart failure. Am J Cardiol 48:934–938, 1981.
31. Lowenthal DT, Dickerman D, Saris SD, Falkner B, Hare TW: The effect of pharmacological interaction on central and peripheral alpha-receptors and pressor response to static exercise. Ann Sports Med 1(3):100–104, 1984.
32. Manhem P, Bramnert M, Hulthen UL, Hokfelt B: The effect of captopril on catecholamines, renin activity, angiotensin II and aldosterone in plasma during physical exercise in hypertensive patients. Eur J Clin Invest 11:389–395, 1981.
33. Fagard R, Lijnen P, Amery A: Hemodynamic response to captopril at rest and during exercise in hypertensive patients. Am J Cardiol 49:1569–1571, 1982.
34. Fagard R, Amery A, Reybrouck T, Lijnen P, Moerman E, et al: Effects of angiotensin antagonism on hemodynamics, renin and catecholamines during exercise. J Appl Physiol 43:440–444, 1977.

35. Stone PH, Antman EM, Muller JE, Braunwald E: Calcium channel blocking agents in the treatment of cardiovascular disorders. Part II: Hemodynamic effects of clinical applications. Ann Intern Med 93:886–904, 1980.
36. Stein DT, Lowenthal DT, Porter RS, Falkner B, Bravo EL, Hare TW: Effects of nifedipine and verapamil on isometric and dynamic exercise in normal subjects. Am J Cardiol 54:386–389, 1984.
37. Subramanian B, Bowles MJ, Davies AB, Raftery EB: Combined therapy with verapamil and propranolol in chronic stable angina. Am J Cardiol 49:125–132, 1982.
38. Moskowitz RM, Piccini PA, Nacarelli G, Selis R: Nifedipine therapy for stable angina pectoris: Preliminary results of effects on angina frequency and treadmill exercise response. Am J Cardiol 44:811–816, 1979.
39. Bonow RO, Leon MB, Rosing DR, Kent KM, Lipson LC, et al: Effects of verapamil and propranolol on left ventricular function and diastolic filling in patients with coronary artery disease: Radionuclide angiographic studies at rest and during exercise. Circulation 65:1337–1350, 1982.
40. Goldstein RE, Rosing DR, Redwood DR, Beiser GD, Epstein SE: Clinical and circulatory effects of isosorbide dinitrate: Comparison with nitroglycerine. Circulation 43:629–640, 1971.
41. Sorensen SG, Ritchie JL, Caldwell JH, Hamilton GW, Kennedy JW: Serial exercise radionuclide angiography. Validation of count-derived changes in cardiac output and quantitation of maximal exercise ventricular volume change after nitroglycerine and propranolol in normal men. Circ 61(3):600–609, 1980.
42. Franciosa JA, Goldsmith SR, Cohn JN: Contrasting immediate and long-term effects of isosorbide dinitrate on exercise capacity in congestive heart failure. Am J Med 69:559–566, 1980.
43. Lee G, Mason DT, Amsterdam E, DeMaria A, Davis VC: Improved exercise tolerance for six hours following isosorbide dinitrate capsules in patients with ischemic heart disease (Abstract). Am J Cardiol 37:150, 1976.
44. Williams MH Jr, Zohman LR, Ratner AC: Hemodynamic effects of cardiac glycosides on normal human subjects during rest and exercise. J Appl Physiol 13:417–421, 1958.
45. Gross GJ, Warltier DC, Hardman HF, Somani P: The effect of ouabain on nutritional circulation and regional myocardial blood flow. Am Heart J 93:487–495, 1977.
46. Parker JO, West RO Jr, Ledwich JR, DiGiorgi S: The effect of acute digitalization on the hemodynamic response to exercise in coronary artery disease. Circulation 40:453–462, 1969.
47. Glancy DL, Higgs LM, O'Brien KP, Epstein SE: Effects of ouabain on the left ventricular response to exercise in patients with angina pectoris. Circulation 43:45–57, 1971.
48. Gooch AS, Natarajan G, Goldberg H: Influence of exercise on arrhythmias induced by digitalis-diuretic therapy in patients with atrial fibrillation. Am J Cardiol 33:230–237, 1974.
49. Gey GO, Levy RH, Fisher L, Pettet G, Bruce RA: Plasma concentration of procainamide and prevalence of exertional arrhythmias. Ann Intern Med 80:718–722, 1974.
50. Gey GO, Levy RH, Pettet G, Fisher L: Quinidine plasma concentration and exertional arrhythmia. Am Heart J 90:19–24, 1975.
51. Surawicz B, Lasseter KC: Effects of drugs on the electrocardiogram. Prog Cardiovasc Dis 13:26–55, 1970.
52. Freedberg AS, Riseman JEF, Speigel ED: Objective evidence of the efficiency of medical therapy in angina pectoris. Am Heart J 22:494–518, 1941.
53. Venerando A: Doping: Pathology and ways to control it. Med Dello Spt 3:972–993, 1963.
54. Costill DL, Dalsky G, Fink W: Effects of caffeine ingestion on metabolism and exercise performance. Med Sci Sports 10:155–158, 1978.
55. Grollman A: The action of alcohol, caffeine and tobacco on the cardiac output (and its related functions) of normal man. J Pharmacol Exp Ther 39:313–327, 1930.
56. Rivers W, Webber H: The action of caffeine on the capacity for muscular work. J Physiol 36:33–47, 1907.

57. Schirlitz K: Uber caffein bei verminderne muskelarbeit. Inter Zeit Ang Physiol Einsch Arbeit 2:273–277, 1930.
58. Axelrod J, Reichenthal J: The fate of caffeine in man and a method for its estimation in biological material. J Pharmacol Exp Ther 107:519–523, 1953.
59. Van Handel PJ, Burke E, Costill DL, Cote R: Physiological responses to cola ingestion. Res Q 48:436–444, 1977.
60. Goldstein A, Warren R, Kaizer S: Psychotropic effects of caffeine in man. I. Interindividual differences in sensitivity to caffeine-induced wakefulness. J Pharmacol Exp Ther 149:156–159, 1965.
61. Essig D, Costill DL, Van Handel PJ: Effects of caffeine ingestion on utilization of muscle glycogen and lipid during leg ergometer cycling. Int J Sports Med 1:86–90, 1980.
62. Robertson D, Johnson GA, Robertson RM, Nies AS, Shand DG, Oates JA: Comparative assessment of stimuli that release neuronal and adrenomedullary catecholamines in man. Circulation 59:637–643, 1979.
63. Victor BS, Lubetsky M, Greden JF: Somatic manifestations of caffeinism. J Clin Psychol 42:185–188, 1981.
64. Regan TJ, Weisse AB, Moschos CB, et al: The myocardial effects of acute and chronic usage of ethanol in man. Trans Assoc Am Physicians 78:282–291, 1965.
65. Regan TJ, Weisse AB, Moschos CB, et al: The myocardial effects of acute and chronic usage of ethanol in man. Trans Assoc Am Physicians 78:282–291, 1965.
66. Conway N: Haemodynamic effects of ethyl alcohol in patients with coronary heart disease. Br Heart J 30:638–644, 1968.
67. Gillespie JA: Vasodilator properties of alcohol. Br Med J 29(2):274–277, 1967.
68. Fewings JD, Hanna MJD, Walsh JA, et al: The effects of ethyl alcohol on the blood vessels of the hand and in man. Br J Pharmacol 27:93–106, 1966.
69. Riff DP, Jain AC, Doyle JT: Acute hemodynamic effects of ethanol on normal human volunteers. Am Heart J 78:592–597, 1969.
70. Blomquist G, Saltin B, Mitchell JH: Acute effects of ethanol ingestion on the response to submaximal and maximal exercise in man. Circulation 42:463–470, 1970.
71. Smith GM, Beecher HK: Amphetamine sulfate and athletic performance. JAMA 170:542, 1959.
72. Karpovich PV: Effect of amphetamine sulfate on athletic performance. JAMA 170:558, 1959.
73. Underwood J: Brutality: Part 3. Speed is all the rage. Sports Illustrated, Aug 28, 1978, p. 20.
74. Kannel WB, Doyle JD, McNamara PM, Quickenton P, Gordon T: Precursors of sudden coronary death. Circulation 51:606–613, 1975.
75. Herbert WH: Cigarette smoking and arteriographically demonstratable coronary artery disease. Chest 67:49–52, 1975.
76. Zalokar JB, Richard JL, Claude JR: Leukocyte count, smoking and myocardial infarction. N Engl J Med 304:465–468, 1981.
77. MacDougall JM, Dembroski TM, Slaats S, Herd JA, Eliot RS: Selective cardiovascular effects of stress and cigarette smoking. J Human Stress 9:13–21, 1983.
78. Gilbert DA: Paradoxical tranquilizing and emotion reducing effects of nicotine. Psychol Bull 86:643–661, 1979.
79. Tashkin DP (moderator): Cannabis 1977. Ann Intern Med 89:539–549, 1978.
80. Gash A, Karliner JS, Janowsky D, Lake LR: Effects of smoking marijuana on left ventricular performance and plasma norepinephrine. Ann Intern Med 89:448–452, 1978.

APPENDIX

AMERICAN COLLEGE OF SPORTS MEDICINE POSITION STAND ON THE USE OF ANABOLIC-ANDROGENIC STEROIDS IN SPORTS*

Based on a comprehensive literature survey and a careful analysis of the claims concerning the ergogenic effects and the adverse effects of anabolic-androgenic steroids, it is the position of the American College of Sports Medicine that:

1. Anabolic-androgenic steroids in the presence of an adequate diet can contribute to increases in body weight, often in the lean mass compartment.
2. The gains in muscular strength achieved through high-intensity exercise and proper diet can be increased by the use of anabolic-androgenic steroids in some individuals.
3. Anabolic-androgenic steroids do not increase aerobic power or capacity for muscular exercise.
4. Anabolic-androgenic steroids have been associated with adverse effects on the liver, cardiovascular system, reproductive system, and psychological status in therapeutic trials and in limited research on athletes. Until further research is completed, the potential hazards of the use of the anabolic-androgenic steroids in athletes must include those found in therapeutic trials.
5. The use of anabolic-androgenic steroids by athletes is contrary to the rules and ethical principles of athletic competition as set forth by many of the sports governing bodies. The American College of Sports Medicine supports these ethical principles and deplores the use of anabolic-androgenic steroids by athletes.

This document is a revision of the 1977 position stand of the American College of Sports Medicine concerning anabolic-androgenic steroids.[4]

BACKGROUND

In 1935 the long-suspected positive effect of androgens on protein anabolism was documented.[56] Subsequently, this effect was confirmed,[53, 77] and the development of 19-nortestosterone heralded the synthesis of

---

steroids that have greater anabolic properties than natural testosterone but less of its virilizing effect.[39] The use of androgenic steroids by athletes began in the early 1950s[106] and has increased through the years, [60, 62, 83, 98, 104, 106] despite warnings about potential adverse reactions[4, 83, 106, 112] and the banning of these substances by sports governing bodies.

ANABOLIC-ANDROGENIC STEROIDS, BODY COMPOSITION AND ATHLETIC PERFORMANCE

Body Composition. Animal studies investigating the effect of anabolic-androgenic steroids on body composition have shown increases in lean body mass, nitrogen retention and muscle growth in castrated males[37, 57, 58] and normal females.[26, 37, 71] The effects of anabolic-androgenic steroids on the body weights of normal, untrained, male animals,[37, 40, 71, 105, 114] treadmill-trained[43, 97] or isometrically-trained rats,[82] or strength-trained monkeys[80] have been minimal to absent; however, the effects of steroids on animals undergoing heavy resistance training have not been adequately studied. Human males who are deficient in natural androgens by castration or other causes have shown significant increases in nitrogen retention and muscular development with anabolic-androgenic steroid therapy.[23, 58, 103] Human males and females involved in experimental[38] and therapeutic trials of anabolic steroids[15, 16, 93] have shown increases in body weight.

The majority of the strength-training studies in which body weight was reported showed greater increases in weight under steroid treatment than under placebo.[17, 41, 42, 50, 61, 74, 94, 96, 107] Other training studies have reported no significant changes in body weight.[21, 27, 31, 34, 100, 108] The weight gained was determined to be lean body mass in three studies that made this determination with hydrostatic weighing techniques.[41, 42, 107] Four other studies found no significant differences in lean body mass between steroid and placebo treatments,[17, 21, 27, 34] but in two of those the mean differences favored the steroid treatment.[21, 27] The extent to which increased water retention accounts for steroid-induced changes in body composition is controversial[17, 42] and has yet to be resolved.

In summary, anabolic-androgenic steroids can contribute to an increase in body weight in the lean mass compartment of the body. The amount of weight gained in the training studies has been small but statistically significant.

Muscular Strength. Strength is an important factor in many athletic events. The literature concerning the efficacy of anabolic steroids for promoting strength development is controversial. Many factors contribute to the development of strength, including heredity, intensity of training, diet, and the status of the psyche.[112] It is very difficult to control all of these factors in an experimental design. The additional variable of dosage is included when drug research is undertaken. Some athletes claim that doses greater than therapeutic are necessary for strength gains[106] even though positive results have been reported using therapeutic (low-dose) regimens.[50, 74, 94, 107] Double-blind studies using anabolic-androgenic steroids are also difficult to conduct because of the physical and/or psychological effects of the drug that, for example, allowed 100% of the participants in one "double-blind" study to correctly identify the steroid phase of the experiment.[32] The placebo effect has been shown to be a factor in studies of anabolic-androgenic steroids as in all drug studies.[6]

In animal studies, the combination of anabolic-androgenic steroids and overload training has not produced larger gains in force production than training alone.[80, 97] However, steroid-induced gains in strength have been reported in experienced[42, 74, 94, 107] and inexperienced weight trainers[50, 51, 96] with[50, 51, 74, 94] and without dietary control or supplemental protein.[42, 96] In contrast, no positive effect of steroids on gains in strength over those produced by training alone were reported in other studies involving experienced[21, 34, 54] and inexperienced weight trainers[17, 27, 31, 41, 54, 61, 100, 108] with[21, 34, 61, 100] and without dietary control or supplemental protein.[17, 27, 31, 41, 54, 108] The studies that reported no changes in strength with anabolic-androgenic steroids have been criticized[112] for the use of inexperienced weight trainers, lack of dietary control,, low-intensity training,[17, 27, 31, 61] and nonspecific testing of strength.[21] The studies that have shown strength gains with the use of anabolic-androgenic steroids have been criticized[83] for inadequate numbers of subjects,[74, 94, 107] improper statistical designs, inadequate execution, and the unsatisfactory reporting of experimental results.

There have been no studies of the effects of the massive doses of steroids used by some athletes over periods of several years. Similarly, there have been no studies of the use of anabolic-androgenic steroids and training in women or children. Theoretically, anabolic and androgenic effects would be greater in women and children because they have naturally lower levels of androgens than men.

Three proposed mechanisms for the actions of the anabolic-androgenic steroids for increases in muscle strength are:

1. Increase in protein synthesis in the muscle as a direct action of the anabolic-androgenic steroid.[81, 82, 92]
2. Blocking of the catabolic effect of glucocorticoids after exercise by increasing the amount of anabolic-androgenic hormone available.[1, 92, 112]
3. Steroid-induced enhancement of aggressive behavior that promotes a greater quantity and quality of weight training.[14]

In spite of the controversial and sometimes contradictory results of the studies in this area, it can be concluded that the use of anabolic-androgenic steroids, especially by experienced weight trainers, can often increase strength gains beyond those seen with training and diet alone. This positive effect on strength is usually small and obviously is not exhibited by all individuals. The explanation for this variability in steroid effects is unclear. When small increments in strength occur, they can be important in athletic competition.

Aerobic Capacity. The effect of anabolic-androgenic steroids on aerobic capacity has also been questioned. The potential of these drugs to increase total blood volume and hemoglobin[88] might suggest a positive effect of steroids on aerobic capacity. However, only three studies indicated positive effects,[3, 51, 54] and there has been no substantiation of these results in subsequent studies.[27, 41, 50, 52] Thus, the majority of evidence shows no positive effect of anabolic-androgenic steroids on aerobic capacity over aerobic training alone.

ADVERSE EFFECTS

Anabolic-androgenic steroids have been associated with many undesirable or adverse effects in laboratory studies and therapeutic trials. The effects of major concern are those on the liver, cardiovascular, and reproductive systems, and on the psychological status of individuals who are using the anabolic-androgenic steroids.

Adverse Effects on the Liver. Impaired excretory function of the liver, resulting in jaundice, has been associated with anabolic-androgenic steroids in a number of therapeutic trials.[76, 84, 90] The possible cause-and-effect nature of this association is strengthened by the observation of jaundice remission after discontinuance of the drug.[76, 84] In studies of athletes using anabolic-androgenic steroids (65 athletes tested),[89, 98, 104] no evidence of cholestasis has been found.

Structural changes in the liver following anabolic steroid treatment have been found in animals[95, 101] and in humans.[73, 86] Conclusions concerning the clinical significance of these changes on a short- or long-term basis have not been drawn. Investigations in athletes for these changes have not been performed, but there is no reason to believe that the athlete using anabolic-androgenic steroids is immune from these effects of the drugs.

The most serious liver complications associated with anabolic-androgenic steroids are peliosis hepatis (blood-filled cysts in the liver of unknown etiology) and liver tumors. Cases of peliosis hepatis have been reported in individuals treated with anabolic-androgenic steroids for various conditions.[7-10, 13, 35, 65, 66, 70, 88, 102] Rupture of the cysts or liver failure resulting from the condition was fatal in some individuals.[9, 70, 102] In other case reports the condition was an incidental finding at autopsy.[8, 10, 66] The possible cause-and-effect nature of the association between peliosis hepatis and the use of anabolic-androgenic steroids is strengthened by the observation of improvement in the condition after discontinuance of drug therapy in some cases.[7, 35] There are no reported cases of this condition in athletes using anabolic-androgenic steroids, but investigations specific for this disorder have not been performed in athletes.

Liver tumors have been associated with the use of anabolic-androgenic steroids in individuals receiving these drugs as a part of their treatment regimen.[28, 29, 49, 67, 69, 99, 115] These tumors are generally benign,[29, 67, 69, 115] but there have been malignant lesions associated with individuals using these drugs.[28, 99, 115] The possible cause-and-effect nature of this association between the use of the drug and tumor development is strengthened by a report of tumor regression after cessation of drug treatment.[49] The 17-alpha-alkylated compounds are the specific family of anabolic steroids indicted in the development of liver tumors.[46, 49] There is one reported case of a 26-year-old male body builder who died of liver cancer after having abused a variety of anabolic steroids for at least four years.[75] The testing necessary for discovery of these tumors is not commonly performed, and it is possible that other tumors associated with steroid use by athletes have gone undetected.

Blood tests of liver function have been reported to be unchanged with steroid use in some training studies[31, 41, 54, 94] and abnormal in other training studies[32, 51] and in tests performed on athletes known to be using anabolic-androgenic steroids.[54, 89, 104] However, the lesions of peliosis hepatis and liver tumors do not always result in blood test abnormalities,[8, 28, 29, 49, 67, 115] and some authors state that liver radioisotope scans, ultrasound, or computed tomography scans are needed for diagnosis.[28, 29, 113]

In summary, liver function tests have been shown to be adversely affected by anabolic-androgenic steroids, especially the 17-alpha-alkylated compounds. The short- and long-term consequences of these changes, though potentially hazardous, have yet to be reported in athletes using these drugs.

Adverse Effects on the Cardiovascular System. The steroid-induced changes that may affect the development of cardiovascular disease include hyperinsulinism and altered glucose tolerance,[111] decreased high-density lipoprotein cholesterol levels,[72, 98] and elevated blood pressure.[68] These effects are variable for different individuals in various clinical situations. Triglycerides are lowered by anabolic-androgenic steroids in certain individuals[24, 72] and are increased in others.[18, 78] Histological examinations of myofibrils and mitochondria from cardiac tissue obtained from laboratory animals have shown that administration of anabolic steroids leads to pathological alterations in these structures.[5, 11, 12] The cardiovascular effects of the anabolic-androgenic steroids, though potentially hazardous, need further research before any conclusions can be made.

Adverse Effects on the Male Reproductive System. The effects of the anabolic-androgenic steroids on the male reproductive system are oligospermia (small number of sperm) and azoospermia (lack of sperm in the semen), decreased testicular size, abnormal appearance of testicular biopsy material, and reductions in testosterone and gonadotropic hormones. These effects have been shown in training studies,[19, 41, 100] studies of normal volunteers,[38] therapeutic trials,[44] and studies of athletes who were using anabolic-androgenic steroids.[55, 79, 104] In view of the changes shown in the pituitary-gonadal axis, the dysfunction accounting for these abnormalities is believed to be steroid-induced suppression of gonadotrophin production.[19, 36, 38, 79] The changes in these hormones are ordinarily reversible after cessation of drug treatment, but the long-term effects of altering the hypothalamic-pituitary-gonadal axis remain unknown. However, there is a report of residual abnormalities in testicular morphology of healthy men 6 months after discontinuing steroid use.[38] It has been reported that the metabolism of androgens to estrogenic compounds may lead to gynecomastia in males.[23, 58, 98, 112]

Adverse Effects on the Female Reproductive System. The effects of androgenic steroids on the female reproductive system include reduction in circulating levels of luteinizing hormone, follicle-stimulating hormone, estrogens, and progesterone; inhibition of folliculogenesis and ovulation; and menstrual cycle changes including prolongation of the follicular phase, shortening of the luteal phase, and amenorrhea.[20, 63, 91]

Adverse Effects on Psychological Status. In both sexes, psychological effects of anabolic-androgenic steroids include increases or decreases in libido, mood swings, and aggressive behavior,[38, 98] which is related to plasma testosterone levels.[25, 85] Administration of steroids causes changes in the electroencephalogram similar to those seen with psycho-stimulant drugs.[47, 48] The possible ramifications of uncontrollably aggressive and possible hostile behavior should be considered prior to the use of anabolic-androgenic steroids.

Other Adverse Effects. Other side effects associated with the anabolic-androgenic steroids include: ataxia;[2] premature epiphysial closure in youths;[23, 58, 64, 109 110] virilization in youths and women, including hirsutism,[45] clitoromegaly,[63, 112] and irreversible deepening of the voice;[22, 33] acne; temporal hair recession; and alopecia.[45] These adverse reactions can occur with the use of anabolic-androgenic steroids and are believed to be dependent on the type of steroid, dosage and duration of drug use.[58] There is no method for predicting which individuals are more likely to develop these adverse effects, some of which are potentially hazardous.

THE ETHICAL ISSUE

Equitable competition and fair play are the foundation of athletic competition. If competition is to remain on this foundation, rules are necessary. The International Olympic Committee (IOC) has defined "doping" as "the administration of or the use of a competing athlete of any substance foreign to the body or of any physiological substance taken in abnormal quantity or taken by an abnormal route of entry into the body, with the sole intention of increasing in an artificial and unfair manner his performance in competition." Accordingly, the medically unjustified use of anabolic steroids with the intention of gaining an athletic advantage is clearly unethical. Anabolic-androgenic steroids are listed as banned substances by the IOC in accordance with the rules against doping. The American College of Sports Medicine supports the position that the eradication of anabolic-androgenic steroid use by athletes is in the best interest of sport and endorses the development of effective procedures for drug detection and of policies that exclude from competition those athletes who refuse to abide by the rules.

The "win at all cost" attitude that has pervaded society places the athlete in a precarious situation. Testimonial evidence suggests that some athletes would risk serious harm and even death if they could obtain a drug that would ensure their winning an Olympic gold medal. However, the use of anabolic-androgenic steroids by athletes is contrary to the ethical principles of athletic competition and is deplored.

REFERENCES

1. Aakvaag, A., O. Bentdol, K. Quigstod, P. Walstod, H. Renningen, and F. Fonnum. Testosterone and testosterone binding globulin (TeBg) in young men during prolonged stress. Int. J. Androl. 1:22–31, 1978.
2. Agrawal, B. L. Ataxia caused by fluoxymesterone therapy in breast cancer. Arch. Intern. Med. 141:953–959, 1981.
3. Albrecht, H. and E. Albrecht. Ergometric, rheographic, reflexographic and electrographic tests at altitude and effects of drugs on human physical performance. Fed. Proc. 28:1262–1267, 1969.
4. American College of Sports Medicine. Position statement on the use and abuse of anabolic-androgenic steroids in sports. Med. Sci. Sports 9(4):xi–xiii, 1977.
5. Appell, H.-J., B. Heller-Umpfenbach, M. Feraudi, and H. Weicker. Ultrastructural and morphometric investigations on the effects of training and administration of anabolic steroids on the myocardium of guinea pigs. Int. J. Sports Med. 4:268–274, 1983.
6. Ariel, G. and W. Saville. Anabolic steroids: the physiological effects of placebos. Med. Sci. Sports 4:124–126, 1972.
7. Arnold, G. L., and M. M. Kaplan. Peliosis hepatis due to oxymetholone—a clinically benign disorder. Am. J. Gastroenterol. 71:213–216, 1979.
8. Asano, A., H. Wakasa, S. Kaise, T. Nishimaki, and R. Kasukawa. Peliosis hepatis. Report on two autopsy cases with a review of literature. Acta Pathol. Jpn. 32:861–877, 1982.
9. Bagheri, S. and J. Boyer. Peliosis hepatis associated with androgenic-anabolic steroid therapy—a severe form of hepatic injury. Ann. Intern. Med. 81:610–618, 1974.
10. Bank, J. I., D. Lykkebo, and I. Hagerstrand. Peliosis hepatis in a child. Acta Ped. Scand. 67:105–107, 1978.
11. Behrendt, H. Effect of anabolic steroid on rat heart muscle cells. I. Intermediate filaments. Cell Tissue Res. 180:305–315, 1977.
12. Behrendt, H. and H. Boffin. Myocardial cell lesions caused by anabolic hormone. Cell Tissue Res. 181:423–426, 1977.
13. Benjamin, D. C. and B. Shunk. A fatal case of peliosis of the liver and spleen. Am. J. Dis. Child. 132:207–208, 1978.
14. Brooks, R. V. Anabolic steroids and athletes. Phys. Sportsmed. 8(3):161–163, 1980.
15. Buchwald, D., S. Argyres, R. E. Easterling, et al. Effects of Nandrolone Decanoate on the anemia of chronic hemodialysis patients. Nephron 18:232–238, 1977.
16. Carter, C. H. The anabolic steroid, Stanozolol, its evaluation in debilitated children. Clin. Pediatr. 4:671–680, 1965.
17. Casner, S. W., R. G. Early, and B. R. Carlson. Anabolic steroid effects on body composition in normal young men. J. Sports Med. Phys. Fitness 11:98–103, 1971.
18. Choi, E. S. K., T. Chung, R. S. Morrison, C. Myers, and M. S. Greenberg. Hypertriglyceridemia in hemodialysis patients during oral dromostanolone therapy for anemia. Am. J. Clin. Nutr. 27:901–904, 1974.
19. Clerico, A., M. Ferdeghini, C. Palombo, et al. Effects of anabolic treatment on the serum levels of gonadotropins, testosterone, prolactin, thyroid hormones and myoglobin of male athletes under physical training. J. Nuclear Med. Allied Sci. 25:79–88, 1981.
20. Cox. D. W., W. L. Heinrichs, C. A. Paulsen, et al. Perturbations of the human menstrual cycle by oxymetholone. Am J. Obstet. Gynecol. 121:121–126, 1975.
21. Crist, D. M., P. J. Stackpole, and G. T. Peake. Effects of androgenic-anabolic steroids on neuromuscular power and body composition. J. Appl. Physiol. 54:366–370, 1983.

22. Damste, P. H. Voice change in adult women caused by virilizing agents. J. Speech Hear. Disord. 32:126–132, 1967.

23. Dorfman, R. I. and R. A. Shipley. Androgens: Biochemistry, Physiology and Clinical Significance. New York: J. Wiley and Sons, 1956.

24. Doyle, A. E., N. B. Pinkus, and J. Green. The use of oxandrolone in hyperlipidaemia. Med. J. Australia 1:127–129, 1974.

25. Ehrenkranz, J., E. Bliss, and M. H. Sheard. Plasma testosterone correlation with aggressive behavior and social dominance in man. Psychosom. Med. 36:469–475, 1974.

26. Exner, G. U., H. W. Staudte, and D. Pette. Isometric training of rats—effects upon fast and slow muscle and modification by an anabolic hormone (Nandrolone Decanoate) I. Female rats. Pflügers Arch. 345:1–14, 1973.

27. Fahey, T. D. and C. H. Brown. The effects of an anabolic steroid on the strength, body composition and endurance of college males when accompanied by a weight training program. Med. Sci. Sports 5:272–276, 1973.

28. Falk, H., L. Thomas, H. Popper, and H. G. Ishak. Hepatic angiosarcoma associated with androgenic-anabolic steroids. Lancet 2:1120–1123, 1979.

29. Farrell, G. C., D. E. Joshua, R. F. Uren, P. J. Baird, K. W. Perkins, and H. Kronenberg. Androgen-induced hepatoma. Lancet 1:430, 1975.

30. Forsyth, B. T. The effect of testosterone propionate at various protein calorie intakes in malnutrition after trauma. J. Lab. Clin. Med. 43:732–740, 1954.

31. Fowler, W. M., Jr., G. W. Gardner, and G. H. Egstrom. Effect of an anabolic steroid on physical performance in young men. J. Appl. Physiol. 20:1038–1040, 1965.

32. Freed, D. L., A. J. Banks, D. Longson, and D. M. Burley. Anabolic steroids in athletics: crossover double-blind trial on weightlifters. Br. Med. J. 2:471–473, 1975.

33. Gelder, L. V. Psychosomatic aspects of endocrine disorders of the voice. J. Commun. Disord. 7:257–262, 1974.

34. Golding, L. A., J. E. Freydinger, and S. S. Fishel. The effect of an androgenic-anabolic steroid and a protein supplement on size, strength, weight and body composition in athletes. Phys. Sportsmed. 2(6):39–45, 1974.

35. Groos, G., O. H. Arnold, and G. Brittinger. Peliosis hepatis after long-term administration of oxymetholone. Lancet 1:874, 1974.

36. Harkness, R. A., B. H. Kilshaw, and B. M. Hobson. Effects of large doses of anabolic steroids. Br. J. Sports Med. 9:70–73, 1975.

37. Heitzman, R. J. The effectiveness of anabolic agents in increasing rate of growth in farm animals; report on experiments in cattle. In: Anabolic Agents in Animal Production, F. C. Lu and J. Rendell (Eds.) Stuttgart: Georg Thieme Publishers, 1976, pp. 89–98.

38. Heller, C. G., D. J. Moore, C. A. Paulsen, W. O. Nelson, and W. M. Laidlaw. Effects of progesterone and synthetic progestins on the reproductive physiology of normal men. Fed. Proc. 18:1057–1065, 1959.

39. Hershberger, J. G., E. G. Shipley, and R. K. Meyer. Myotrophic activity of 19-nortestosterone and other steroids determined by modified levator ani muscle method. Proc. Soc. Exper. Biol. Med. 83:175–180, 1953.

40. Hervey, G. R. and I. Hutchinson. The effects of testosterone on body weight and composition in the rat. J. Endocrinol. 57:xxiv–xxv, 1973.

41. Hervey, G. R., I. Hutchinson, A. V. Knibbs, et al. Anabolic effects of methandienone in men undergoing athletic training. Lancet 2:699–702, 1976.

42. Hervey, G. R., A. V. Knibbs, L. Burkinshaw, et al. Effects of methandienone on the performance and body composition of men undergoing athletic training. Clin. Sci. 60:457–461, 1981.

43. Hickson, R. C., W. W. Heusner, W. D. Van Huss, et al. Effects of Diabanol and high-intensity sprint training on body composition of rats. Med. Sci. Sports 8:191–195, 1976.

44. Holma, P. and H. Aldercreutz. Effect of an anabolic steroid (metandienon) on plasma LH, FSH, and testosterone and on the response to intravenous administration of LRH. Acta Endocrinol. 83:856–864, 1976.

45. Houssay, A. B. Effects of anabolic-androgenic steroids on the skin including hair and

sebaceous glands. In: Anabolic-Androgenic Steroids, C. D. Kochakan (Ed.). New York: Springer-Verlag, 1976, pp. 155–190.

46. Ishak, K. G. Hepatic lesions caused by anabolic and contraceptive steroids. Sem. Liver Dis. 1:116–128, 1981.

47. Itil, T. M. Neurophysiological effects of hormones in humans: computer EEG profiles of sex and hypothalamic hormones. In: Hormones, Behavior and Psychotherapy, E J. Sachar (Ed.). New York: Raven Press, 1976, pp. 31–40.

48. Itil, T. M., R. Cora, S. Akpinar, W. M. Herrmann, and C. J. Patterson. Psychotropic action of sex hormones: computerized EEG in establishing the immediate CNS effects of steroid hormones. Curr. Ther. Res. 16:1147–1170, 1974.

49. Johnson, F. L., K. G. Lerner, M. Siegel, et al. Association of androgenic-anabolic steroid therapy with development of hepatocellular carcinoma. Lancet 2:1273, 1972.

50. Johnson, L. C., G. Fisher, L. J. Silvester, and C. C. Hofheins. Anabolic steroid: effects of strength, body weight, oxygen uptake and spermatogenesis upon mature males. Med. Sci. Sports 4:43–45, 1972.

51. Johnson, L. C. and J. P. O'Shea. Anabolic steroid: effects on strength development. Science 164:957–959, 1969.

52. Johnson, L. C., E. S. Roundy, P. E. Allsen, A. G. Fisher, and L. J. Silvester. Effect of anabolic steroid treatment on endurance. Med. Sci. Sports 7:287–289, 1975.

53. Kenyon, A. T., K. Knowlton, and I. Sandiford. The anabolic effects of the androgens and somatic growth in man. Ann. Intern. Med. 20:632–654, 1944.

54. Keul, J., H. Deus, and W. Kinderman. Anabole hormone: Schadigung, Leistungsfahigkeit und Stoffwechses. Med. Klin. 71:497–503, 1976.

55. Kilshaw, B. H., R. A. Harkness, B. M. Hobson, and A. W. M. Smith. The effects of large doses of the anabolic steroid, methandrostenolone, on an athlete. Clin. Endocrinol. 4:537–541, 1975.

56. Kochakian, C. D. and J. R. Murlin. The effect of male hormones on the protein and energy metabolism of castrate dogs. J. Nutr. 10:437–458, 1935.

57. Kochakian, C. D. and B. R. Endahl. Changes in body weight of normal and castrated rats by different doses of testosterone propionate. Proc. Soc. Exper. Biol. Med. 100:520–522, 1959.

58. Kruskemper, H. L. Anabolic Steroids. New York: Academic Press, 1968, pp. 128–133, 162–164, 182.

59. Landau, R. L. The metabolic effects of anabolic steroids in man. In: Anabolic-Androgenic Steroids, C. D. Kochakian (Ed.). New York: Springer-Verlag, 1976, pp. 45–72.

60. Ljungqvist, A. The use of anabolic steroids in top Swedish athletes. Br. J. Sports Med. 9:82, 1975.

61. Loughton, S. J. and R. O. Ruhling. Human strength and endurance responses to anabolic steroid and training. J. Sports Med. 17:285–296, 1977.

62. MacDougall, J. D., D. G. Sale, G. C. B. Elder, and J. R. Sutton, Muscle ultrastructural characteristics of elite powerlifters and bodybuilders. Eur. J. Applied Physiol. 48:117–126, 1982.

63. Maher, J. M., E. L. Squires, J. L. Voss, and R. K. Shideler. Effect of anabolic steroids on reproductive function of young mares. J. Am. Vet. Med. Assoc. 183:519–524, 1983.

64. Mason, A. S. Male precocity: the clinician's view. In: The Endocrine Function of the Human Testis, V. H. T. James, M. Serra, and L. Martini (Eds.). New York: Academic Press, 1974, pp. 131–143.

65. McDonald, E. C. and C. E. Speicher. Peliosis hepatis associated with administration of oxymetolone. JAMA 240:243–244, 1978.

66. McGiven, A. R. Peliosis hepatis: case report and review of pathogenesis. J. Pathol. 101:283–285, 1970.

67. Meadows, A. T., J. L. Naiman, and M. Valdes-Dapena. Hepatoma associated with androgen therapy for aplastic anemia. J. Pediatr. 85:109–110, 1974.

68. Messerli, F. H. and E. D. Frohlich. High blood pressure: a side effect of drugs, poisons, and food. Arch. Intern. Med. 139:682–687, 1979.

69. Mulvihill, J. J., R. L. Ridolfi, F. R. Schultz, M. S. Brozy, and P. B. T. Haughton. Hepatic

adenoma in Fanconi anemia treated with oxymetholone. J. Pediatr. 87:122–124, 1975.

70. Nadell, J. and J. Kosek. Peliosis hepatis. Arch. Pathol. Lab. Med. 101:405–410, 1977.
71. Nesheim, M. C. Some observations on the effectiveness of anabolic agents in increasing the growth rate of poultry. In: Anabolic Agents in Animal Production, F. C. Lu and J. Rendel (Eds.). Stuttgart: Georg Thieme Publishers, 1976, pp. 110–114.
72. Olsson, A. G., L. Oro, and S. Rossner. Effects of oxandrolone on plasma lipoproteins and the intravenous fat tolerance in man. Atherosclerosis 19:337–346, 1974.
73. Orlandi, F., A. Jezequel, and A. Melliti. The action of some anabolic steroids on the structure and the function of human liver cell. Tijdschr. Gastro-Enterol. 7:109–113, 1964.
74. O'Shea, J. P. The effects of an anabolic steroid on dynamic strength levels of weightlifters. Nutr. Rep. Int. 4:363–370, 1971.
75. Overly, W. L., J. A. Dankoff, B. K. Wang, and U. D. Singh. Androgens and hepatocellular carcinoma in an athlete. Ann Intern. Med. 100:158–159, 1984.
76. Palva, I. P. and C. Wasastjerna. Treatment of aplastic anaemia with methenolone. Acta Haematol. 47:13–20, 1972.
77. Papanicolaou, G. N. and G. A. Falk. General muscular hypertrophy induced by androgenic hormone. Science 87:238–239, 1938.
78. Reeves, R. D., M. D. Morris, and G. L. Barbour. Hyperlipidemia due to oxymetholone therapy. JAMA 236:464–472, 1976.
79. Remes, K., P. Vuopio, M. Jarvinen, M. Harkonen, and H. Adlercreutz. Effect of short-term treatment with an anabolic steroid (methandienone) and dehydroepiandrosterone sulphate on plasma hormones, red cell volume and 2,3-diphosphoglycerate in athletes. Scand. J. Clin. Lab. Invest. 37:577–586, 1977.
80. Richardson, J. H. A comparison of two drugs on strength increase in monkeys. J. Sports Med. Phys. Fitness 17:251–254, 1977.
81. Rogozkin, V. A. The role of low molecular weight compounds in the regulation of skeletal muscle genome activity during exercise. Med. Sci. Sports 8:1–4, 1976.
82. Rogozkin, V. A. Anabolic steroid metabolism in skeletal muscle. J. Steroid Biochem. 11:923–926, 1979.
83. Ryan, A. J. Anabolic steroids are fool's gold. Fed. Proc. 40:2682–2688, 1981.
84. Sacks, P., D. Gale, T. H. Bothwell, K. Stevens. Oxymetholone therapy in aplastic and other refractory anaemias. S. Afr. Med. J. 46:1607–1615, 1972.
85. Scaramella, T. J. and W. A. Brown. Serum testosterone and aggressiveness in hockey players. Psychosom. Med. 40:262–265, 1978.
86. Schaffner, F., H. Popper, and V. Perez. Changes in bile canaliculi produced by norethandrolone: electron microscopic study of human and rat liver. J. Lab. Clin. Med. 56:623–628, 1960.
87. Shahidi, N. T. Androgens and erythropoeisis. N. Engl. J. Med. 289:72–80, 1973.
88. Shapiro, P., R. M. Ikedo, B. H. Ruebner, M. H. Conners, C. C. Halsted, and C. F. Abildgaard. Multiple hepatic tumors and peliosis hepatitis in Fanconi's anemia treated with androgens. Am. J. Dis. Child. 131:1104–1106, 1977.
89. Shephard, R. J., D. Killinger, and T. Fried. Responses to sustained use of anabolic steroid. Br. J. Sports Med. 11:170–173, 1977.
90. Skarberg, K. O., L. Engstedt, S. Jameson, et al. Oxymetholone treatment in hypoproliferative anaemia. Acta Haematol. 49:321–330, 1973.
91. Smith, K. D., L. J. Rodriguez-Rigau, R. K. Tcholakian, and E. Steinberg. The relation between plasma testosterone levels and the lengths of phases of the menstrual cycle. Fertil. Steril. 32:403–407, 1979.
92. Snochowski, M., E. Dahlberg, E. Eriksson, and J. A. Gustafsson. Androgen and glucocorticoid receptors in human skeletal muscle cytosol. J. Steroid Biochem. 14:765–771, 1981.
93. Spiers, A. S. D., S. F. DeVita, M. J. Allar, S. Richards, and N. Sedransk. Beneficial effects of an anabolic steroid during cytotoxic chemotherapy for metastatic cancer. J. Med. 12:433–445, 1981.
94. Stamford, B. A. and R. Moffatt. Anabolic steroid: effectiveness as an ergogenic aid to experienced weight trainers. J. Sports Med. Phys. Fitness 14:191–197, 1974.

95. Stang-Voss, C. and H.-J. Appel. Structural alterations of liver parenchyma induced by anabolic steroids. Int. J. Sports Med. 2:101–105, 1981.
96. Steinbach, M. Uber den Einfluss Anaboler wirkstoffe auf Korpergewicht, Muskelkraft und Muskeltraining. Sportarzt Sportmed. 11:485–492, 1968.
97. Stone, M. H., M. E. Rush, and H. Lipner. Responses to intensive training and methandrostenelone administration: II. Hormonal, organ weights, muscle weights and body composition. Pflugers Arch. 375:147–151, 1978.
98. Strauss, R. H., H. E. Wright, G. A. M. Finerman, and D. H. Catlin. Side effects of anabolic steroids in weight-trained men. Phys. Sportsmed. 11(12):87–96, 1983.
99. Stromeyer, F. W., D. H. Smith, and K. G. Ishak. Anabolic steroid therapy and intrahepatic cholangiocarcinoma. Cancer 43:440–443, 1979.
100. Stromme, S. B., H. D. Meen, and A. Aakvaag. Effects of an androgenic-anabolic steroid on strength development and plasma testosterone levels in normal males. Med. Sci. Sports 6:203–208, 1974.
101. Taylor, W., S. Snowball, C. M. Dickson, and M. Lesna. Alterations of liver architecture in mice treated with anabolic androgens and diethylnitrosamine. NATO Adv. Study Inst. Series, Series A 52:279–288, 1982.
102. Taxy, J. B. Peliosis: a morphologic curiosity becomes an iatrogenic problem. Hum. Pathol. 9:331–340, 1978.
103. Tepperman, J. Metabolic and Endocrine Physiology. Chicago: Yearbook Medical Publishers, 1973, p. 70.
104. Thomson, D. P., D. R. Pearson, and D. L. Costill. Use of anabolic steroids by national level athletes. Med. Sci. Sports Exerc. 13:111, 1981. (Abstract)
105. VanderWal, P. General aspects of the effectiveness of anabolic agents in increasing protein production in farm animals, in particular in bull calves. In: Anabolic Agents in Animal Production, F. C. Lu and J. Rendel (Eds.). Stuttgart: Georg Thieme Publishers, 1976, pp. 60–78.
106. Wade, N. Anabolic steroids: doctors denounce them, but athletes aren't listening. Science 176:1399–1403, 1972.
107. Ward, P. The effect of an anabolic steroid on strength and lean body mass. Med. Sci. Sports 5:277–282, 1973.
108. Weiss, V. and H. Muller. Aur Frage der Beeinflussung des Kraft-trainings durch Anabole Hormone. Schweiz. Z. Sportmed. 16:79–89, 1968.
109. Whitelaw, M. J., T. N. Foster, and W. H. Graham. Methandrostenolone (Diabanol): a controlled study of its anabolic and androgenic effect in children. Pediatric. Pharm. Ther. 68:291–296, 1966.
110. Wilson, J. D. and J. E. Griffin. The use and misuse of androgens. Metabolism 29:1278–1295, 1980.
111. Woodard, T. L., G. A. Burghen, A. E. Kitabchi, and J. A. Wilimas. Glucose intolerance and insulin resistance in aplastic anemia treated with oxymetholone. J. Clin. Endocrinol. Metab. 53:905–908, 1981.
112. Wright, J. E. Anabolic steroids and athletes. Exerc. Sport Sci. Rev. 8:149–202, 1980.
113. Yamagishi, M., A. Hiraoka, and H. Uchino. Silent hepatic lesions detected with computed tomography in aplastic anemia patients administered androgens for a long period. Acta Haematol. Jpn. 45:703–710, 1982.
114. Young, M., H. R. Crookshank, and L. Ponder. Effects of an anabolic steroid on selected parameters in male albino rats. Res. Q. 48:653–656, 1977.
115. Zevin, D., H. Turani, A. Cohen, and J. Levi. Androgen-associated hepatoma in a hemodialysis patient. Nephron 29:274–276, 1981.

INDEX

Page numbers in *italics* indicate illustrations. Page numbers followed by t indicate tables.